WHY YOUR
TEETH
MIGHT BE
KILLING YOU

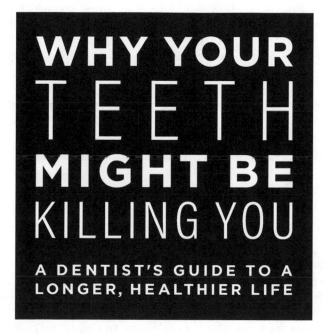

WHY YOUR TEETH MIGHT BE KILLING YOU

A DENTIST'S GUIDE TO A LONGER, HEALTHIER LIFE

DR. STEVEN R. FREEMAN

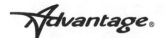

Published by Advantage, Charleston, South Carolina.
Member of Advantage Media Group.

ADVANTAGE is a registered trademark, and the Advantage colophon is a trademark of Advantage Media Group, Inc.

Printed in the United States of America.

10 9 8 7 6 5 4 3 2 1

ISBN: 978-1-59932-879-9
LCCN: 2018939335

Cover design by Melanie Cloth.
Layout design by Carly Blake.

This publication is designed to provide accurate and authoritative information in regard to the subject matter covered. It is sold with the understanding that the publisher is not engaged in rendering legal, accounting, or other professional services. If legal advice or other expert assistance is required, the services of a competent professional person should be sought.

Advantage Media Group is proud to be a part of the Tree Neutral® program. Tree Neutral offsets the number of trees consumed in the production and printing of this book by taking proactive steps such as planting trees in direct proportion to the number of trees used to print books. To learn more about Tree Neutral, please visit **www.treeneutral.com**.

Advantage Media Group is a publisher of business, self-improvement, and professional development books and online learning. We help entrepreneurs, business leaders, and professionals share their Stories, Passion, and Knowledge to help others Learn & Grow. Do you have a manuscript or book idea that you would like us to consider for publishing? Please visit **advantagefamily.com** or call **1.866.775.1696**.

TABLE OF CONTENTS

PART III

DELIVERING QUALITY DENTAL CARE

A WORD FROM
THE AUTHOR

'm sure you've heard the old saying: "An ounce of prevention is worth a pound of cure." Not only is this true of dentistry but, when it comes to dental health, an ounce of prevention could mean your life!

Many readers may think this sounds over the top, but think about it: you have millions of bacteria living in your mouth. Some are actually good for us, but many of them are harmful. Left unchecked, these harmful bacteria, combined with your body's response to them, can lead not only to tooth loss but also to diabetes, heart disease, kidney disease, cancer, and ultimately death. Your dentist can be one of the frontline defenders of your overall health against disease. This is what preventative dental care is all about.

Yet people still don't consider dental care to be as serious as it is. The history of dentistry doesn't help with this. In a sense, dentistry was the first medical specialty, breaking off from the main category of medicine hundreds of years ago. Now, specialization is great—it leads to many advances. But because dentistry has been treated apart from medicine for such a long time, people have almost forgotten that it is a branch of medicine at all. The result is that they neglect dental health, not realizing it is a part of overall body health. If you have a badly damaged or infected leg, for instance, you're most likely going to hurry to the doctor; but the same can't be said of teeth—you may put off treatment, thinking it isn't that important. It's almost like our teeth are second-class organs compared to the rest of our body.

Whether we like it or not, a bacterial infection in your mouth can be just as harmful as one on your leg; and your dentist can be just as instrumental in keeping you healthy—even saving your life—as any other medical doctor can be. In this book, I discuss a number of ways that your dental health has a ripple effect through your whole body, as well as a number of procedures a dentist can do in his or her office that can dramatically increase the length of your life—and make you look better along the way.

After all, dentistry has a cosmetic side too. It would be a mistake, though, to see certain procedures as "merely" cosmetic, as they can make a drastic difference in a person's confidence. We must remember that psychological well-being is an important part of health too. From that point of view, an attractive smile is not a luxury; everyone deserves to smile confidently and live healthily.

While my father was an oral surgeon, I began my career in dentistry with a focus on the cosmetic side of things. I developed skills with a number of procedures (some of which will be discussed in this book) but did not actually find a niche until branching out into general dentistry and circling back around to oral surgery myself, ultimately specializing in placing dental implants. I have now done more implants than my father did in his entire career.

I now see, on a daily basis, the harmful effects of poor oral health. To take a major example: while many people think of implants as a cosmetic matter, having a tooth missing places undue stress on the other teeth, which are increasingly at risk of infection (leading to all of the health effects I mentioned) and further loss. There is a feedback relationship where tooth loss harms the other teeth, leading to more loss and more harm and infection … and so on. So the investment in one tooth, in the form of an implant, is an investment in your other teeth as well.

Likewise, an investment in good dental health is an investment in your overall health. The main focus of this book is the relationship between health and dental care. While this is directly addressed in Part I, it also motivates Part II, which describes what are typically considered more cosmetic procedures but which themselves are major contributors to psychological well-being. Finally, in Part III, I focus more on what I take to be the broader fundamentals of quality dental care—what makes a good dental practice and how I try to exemplify that in my own practice. I share my big-picture approach with other dentists, with my patients, and now with you, in the hopes that all will realize the importance of quality dental care and good dental health in preventing harm on a larger scale down the road—so that we can all smile to live.

PART I

DENTISTRY AS HEALTHCARE

CHAPTER 1

OPEN UP: DENTAL CARE AND BODILY HEALTH

I tell my patients all the time that the teeth and body are part of one big interconnected system. Sometimes they don't believe me. One patient's reaction was, "I thought you were supposed to be a dentist; now you're telling me I should get my blood pressure checked and be tested for diabetes? All you did was poke my gums!" He called me the next day, stunned: "I saw my primary care doctor right after I saw you, and he told me exactly the same thing you did!"

The key thing to understand about general dentistry, and what I emphasize in my own practice, is that mouth health is tied to overall body health. Our mouths are systematically connected in a number of ways to our bodies as a whole and to the functioning of total body systems. It might sound extreme to say, "Hey, the cleaner your teeth are, the less likely you are to die of a heart attack or get diabetes," but it's actually true. Don't forget that your dentist is a medical professional and can serve as a front line of defense against illness if you do your part and maintain good oral health.

WANT TO LEARN MORE ABOUT THE ELITE SMILE EXPERIENCE? CHAPTER 1 COVERS:

- **gum disease**
  - the source of gum disease
  - gingivitis
  - periodontal disease
- **dental care and the immune system**
- **pregnancy and oral health**
- **oral health and diabetes**

RUNAWAY BACTERIA

We clean our teeth—whether it be brushing or going to the dentist for a cleaning—for more than just freshening our breath. We do it to get the bacteria off of our teeth and out of our mouths. Bacteria accumulate in our mouths in the form of plaque, and letting that plaque hang around can have serious negative effects. Most obviously, gum disease results from the irritation that the plaque causes. The National Institute of Health (NIH) estimates that 80 percent of adults have some level of gum disease, ranging from mild gingivitis to advanced periodontal disease.

Each of our teeth sits inside a kind of pocket, and inside that pocket the root of the tooth is connected, by a ligament, to bone. Typically, the root, ligament, and bone are protected by the tight seal of the pocket around the teeth. Plaque, however, sits right at the gum line, which is the edge of the pocket. The mouth—warm, wet, and protected—is the ideal incubator for the bacteria that make up the plaque. These bacteria constantly produce toxins; adding sugar (the bacteria's preferred food source, which is abundant in our diets) is like throwing gasoline on a fire. That's why brushing your teeth and cutting back on sugar are both such important parts of maintaining oral health.

Gum disease is the result of neglecting this kind of oral care. At the least-severe extreme, we have gingivitis, which is simply the inflammation of the gums that results from irritation by the bacteria in plaque. With gingivitis, the gums become inflamed to the point that they become puffy. This inflammation is just the way the body responds to the bacteria sitting along the gums in the form of plaque. If the plaque is not removed, it can harden into what is called "calculus." This calculus up against the gum line just harbors more bacteria, and the inflammation gets worse.

Eventually, the gums are going to get tired of the inflammation and start to move away from the bacteria. In other words, the gums start to recede in order to escape the irritation caused by the bacteria, and that protective pocket begins to loosen. The problem now is that the new spot where the gums sit up against the teeth—closer to the root of the tooth—will again develop more plaque on it if you don't clean your teeth, which leads to more inflammation and more recession and soon a vicious cycle of the gum getting shorter and shorter.

A traditional dental cleaning removes the bacteria and plaque above the gum line. Unfortunately, for some people, this may not be enough. Below the gum line, there lives a group of bacteria called "the red complex," which is linked to periodontal disease. Red complex bacteria can also harden into a calculus, but this time a traditional dental cleaning will not do the trick.

While the bacteria you see on your teeth as plaque are aerobic, meaning they need exposure to oxygen, the red complex bacteria are anaerobic; the further they can get from oxygen, the better. That is why these bacteria live deep below the gum line, so fighting them requires a "deep cleaning" that goes underneath the gum line to remove the calculus and accumulating bacteria.

Different people with different genetics are always going to have different needs when it comes to dental health, and this is no exception. Some people, just because of genetics, have a greater amount of red complex bacteria or have immune systems that do not fight it as well; this means that they are more susceptible to periodontal disease.

Whichever form of bacteria is present, if the infection penetrates deeply enough, it will start eating away at the supporting ligament and bone so that the tooth becomes unstable. This loss of bone support as well as gums around the teeth is called "attachment loss." Periodontal disease is just the result of a vicious cycle that occurs here: the bone continues to recede, the gums keep getting shorter, and thus the support for the teeth becomes less and less and less; at some point, of course, the teeth just start coming out.

Periodontal disease is essentially a runaway infection. It can be localized, but typically it affects the whole mouth. If you have red gums, if your gums hurt, or if they bleed when you brush your teeth, these can be signs of the approach of periodontal disease, and you should seek the help of a dentist immediately.

THE IMMUNE REACTION

If you neglect to see a dentist, or more generally, if you don't clean your teeth, you can basically have a bacterial infection the size of your fist sitting there inside your mouth at all times.

Not only can this lead to tooth loss (in fact, periodontal disease is the number-one reason Americans lose their teeth) but the bacteria can actually move into the bloodstream, potentially worsening other chronic conditions. For example, it is associated with increases in harmful types of cholesterol in the bloodstream and can double your chances of having a heart attack.

> *If you neglect to see a dentist, or more generally, if you don't clean your teeth, you can basically have a bacterial infection the size of your fist sitting there inside your mouth at all times.*

This also leads to a huge immune system reaction. In fact, just the accumulation of plaque can trigger a harmful reaction from our immune system. When tissue is irritated, the immune system signals the liver to release C-reactive protein (CRP), which is a response to inflammation anywhere in the body. Basically, CRP puts the immune system on high alert. If you constantly have bacteria in your mouth, then your liver releases more CRP and your immune system ends up working overtime.

CRP has far-ranging negative effects on the body if it stays in your system too long. For example, it contributes to the stiffening of the arteries and increases the likelihood that they will accumulate plaque. The blood vessels become less flexible, and that, combined with increased clotting (another effect of CRP), means the heart has to work harder, and blockage of the blood vessels becomes more likely. This leads to heart disease (the leading cause of death in the US), heart attacks, and high blood pressure—all of which are associated with high levels of CRP.

For this reason, the more CRP you have in your body, the greater the wear and tear on your immune system and (other things being equal) the less healthy you end up being. This actually does increase your chances of things like heart attacks, strokes, and diabetes. Many medical conditions can be linked to high levels of CRP—even cancer. So again, the cleaner your teeth are, the healthier you end up being overall. It's really important that you get your teeth cleaned to bring down those plaque levels in your mouth.

The immune reaction is particularly significant for pregnant women. Again, it may seem like a stretch—what could the health of your mouth have to do with the health of your unborn child?—but everything is interconnected. The two biggest risks associated with a mother with an unhealthy mouth are preterm delivery and low birth weight—and these are indeed serious risks. Sadly, babies born with low birth weight are twenty times less likely than children born in the typical weight range to reach their first birthday.

About 10 percent of all babies in the US are born preterm. This can lead to numerous health problems throughout life. The time spent in the womb is a time for the baby to develop—it cooks, just like a bun in an oven, as the expression goes. If the bun doesn't stay in the oven long enough, it hasn't cooked enough: the baby will be underdeveloped. Preterm babies will often begin their lives with a stay in the neonatal intensive care unit, due to problems associated with underdeveloped and inadequately functioning heart, intestines, lungs, and eyes. Once the placenta is gone, we have to start treating them like babies, but preterm babies are not ready for that treatment yet.

So preterm babies in general are at much higher risk of serious health problems. But what does this have to do with oral health? Well, the presence of bacteria, as I have mentioned, causes an immune response that basically raises the alarm. These signals, and the antibodies that they create, can cross the placenta and enter the baby's bloodstream. This activates the baby's immune system, which has not fully developed, as it should not have to operate at all while the baby is still in utero. The system is being signaled to go into operation despite the fact that it does not yet know how to operate. The baby's immune response can be severely damaging, as the baby's body does not yet know how to handle it; this, for example, is connected to the development of cerebral palsy.

Of course, the bacteria from the mouth can also, if infection gets bad enough, enter the mother's bloodstream and cross the placenta, at which point the baby has a bacterial infection. All the baby wants to do in the womb is sleep, poop, and grow; added stress means it doesn't develop as well, and bacteria are a serious stressor.

The medical community has made great advances in accepting the "healthy mouth, healthy body" connection but has been very slow to take the next step of linking the oral health of a pregnant woman to the health of her unborn child. Yet the evidence supports this connection. This connection is taken so seriously in my household that my wife had her teeth cleaned every three months when she was pregnant with our two children. When a woman is pregnant, taking good care of her teeth and getting quality dental care are not only important to *her* health but to that of her child as well.

THE LIST GOES ON ...

I have only focused in on some of the main ways that oral health affects the rest of your body, but the interconnections between all of these systems are vast. Your oral health, for instance, can directly affect your kidney health, as well as your lungs. It can even have an impact on your joints; arthritis rates are higher among those who have periodontal disease.

CRP has your immune system on high alert to fight inflammation at all times. This leaves room for cancer cells to develop where they otherwise would not have. This is not just oral cancer (which itself can be deadly) but cancer throughout the body. In fact, people with poor oral health are at much higher risk of lung cancer—even if they are not smokers! In some cases, like this one, the links are not even fully understood, but the correlations are there. To make matters worse, some cancer treatments can actually worsen oral health due to their impact on the immune system, leading to a vicious cycle.

A similarly vicious cycle of worsening oral and bodily health occurs with a condition that is sadly widespread in the US: diabetes. As you may know—especially if you are diabetic yourself—diabetes is an impairment in the body's ability to produce insulin, which regulates the levels of glucose (sugar) in the blood. This leads to very high levels of sugar in the blood. Essentially, with diabetes, the body simply does not transform food into energy as efficiently. This can lead to overeating and poorer nutritional health, including increased sugar intake. This is not only harmful to the teeth, as mentioned, but it also, of course, leads to weight gain and further inefficiency in the body. (Incidentally, this also increases the chances of obstructive sleep apnea, which I discuss in a later chapter.) You can see how this leads to a vicious cycle of deteriorating health.

Diabetes also lowers the body's ability to produce antibodies to fight infection, so the whole cycle of bacteria growth leading to periodontal disease occurs even more rapidly. Some of the damage that the bacteria do to the ligament and bone that support the teeth, for instance, can be counteracted by the body's ability to heal itself. The weakening of this immune response in people with diabetes means that the healing process takes place much more slowly, allowing the periodontal disease to take hold that much more effectively. It is no surprise then that gum disease is highly correlated with diabetes.

Many people with diabetes are used to measuring their blood glucose level on a daily basis and reporting their A1C (i.e. their average blood glucose level over the last ninety days) to their primary care doctor. While it may not occur to them to report this number to their dentist as well, it can be beneficial. Given the tight link between oral health and the bodily conditions that have to be so closely monitored with diabetes, the dentist can assist in forming a front line of defense to keep a diabetic patient healthy. On a related note, pregnant women with poor oral health are at increased risk of gestational diabetes—yet another link between the oral health of a pregnant woman and the health of her unborn child.

Another instance of a systematic connection that is not fully understood is the particularly alarming link between tooth loss and dementia in old age. Not only are people suffering from dementia more likely to lose teeth (due to poor oral health) but people with missing teeth—even a single missing tooth—are at higher risk for developing dementia later in life. Again, the connection is not altogether clear, but this suggests that implants, which are often thought to mainly affect appearance, may not be so cosmetic after all. In fact, there are a lot of reasons to get an implant, whether it's a front or back tooth. While I'll talk more about implants in a later chapter, it's worth noting here that missing teeth put stress on the other teeth, leading to another vicious cycle where having one missing tooth makes it more likely that you will lose others.

TAKING CARE

Hopefully I have made the deep systemic links between oral health and bodily health very clear; the health of your teeth is not secondary to your health and should be taken just as seriously as the health of other parts of your body. What does good dental care and oral health involve, though?

Again, it is a complex system, but good oral health starts with what you put in your mouth. As I mentioned, sugar, in addition to the harmful effects it has on your body as a whole, is just fuel for the growth of the bacteria in your mouth. Avoiding sugar is thus a cornerstone to a mouth-healthy diet. Eating healthily and drinking tea, on the other hand, can have a healing effect on your mouth. Of course, this will all be for nothing if you don't clean your teeth regularly, which involves not just brushing and flossing but seeing a dentist for regular dental care.

CHAPTER 2

BEYOND CLEANING

had a patient, Nate, come to me when, in his words, he "couldn't take the pain anymore."

"When did the pain start?" I asked.

"Oh, about a year ago."

"And when was the last time you came to see me?"

"Oh, that was more like two years ago or so," he said.

I took a look and, sure enough, Nate had several cavities, and I would have to take aggressive action. While the cavities were fairly new, his teeth had been sensitive long before they developed—signaling that there was a problem. The cavities could have been prevented if he had come in more regularly and especially if he had alerted me to the sensitivity problem earlier on.

I asked Nate about his diet. It turned out he was a writer who spent most of his day looking at a computer and sipping on a high-sugar, high-acid soda—a dentist's worst nightmare! That meant the sensitivity could have been prevented with more regular cleanings and, especially, a change in dietary habits.

Cases like Nate's are altogether too common, and, though I would like it if my job as a dentist were just to do regular cleanings, it is cases like these where all the other techniques of general dentistry come into play—call it damage control.

WANT TO LEARN MORE ABOUT THE ELITE SMILE EXPERIENCE? CHAPTER 2 COVERS:

- **tooth sensitivity**
  - causes of sensitivity
  - the role of fluoride
  - clenching and grinding
- **fillings**
- **cutting-edge crowns and ceramics**
  - crowns
  - CEREC technology

WHY SO SENSITIVE?

Many people make the mistake of only consulting a dentist after a problem has gotten way out of hand—for example, when they have developed full-blown periodontal disease or a mouthful of cavities. They may ignore the gum pain or sore tooth, thinking it's not that big of a deal. However, not only is a regular dental cleaning important for all of the reasons I discussed in the previous chapter but you should also consult your dentist at any sign of a problem. Teeth should not hurt or bleed; if they do, it is better to address the problem as early as possible than to put it off.

Take sensitivity, for instance. Tooth sensitivity is a common problem that shouldn't occur and that quality dental care can prevent. While obviously not as severe as periodontal disease, it can have negative effects on your life, from ruining your favorite drink or ice cream to leading you to brush less frequently and, thus, take poorer care of your dental health overall. While common—I find that about one out of three guests in my practice report having tooth sensitivity—it is not normal and should not occur.

Sensitivity occurs because our teeth are porous, and, if they are exposed, those pores act as an expressway to the nerve of your tooth, which causes pain when you have something cold. To address sensitivity, the pores need to be either covered or closed up. Of course, there are plenty of toothpastes out there on the market for people with sensitive teeth, and that is what they do: use fluoride and potassium to close the pores.

Fluoride in particular is beneficial to oral, and thus overall, health. When fluoride attaches to the surface of our teeth, it makes it more difficult for bacteria to adhere to that surface. It also helps seal the pores in your teeth—which means it helps with sensitivity and whitening of the teeth by keeping material that could stain the teeth out of the pores.

That is why places that have fluoride in the drinking water experience greatly reduced numbers of cavities in residents—it unquestionably helps teeth. Of course, too much fluoride in the drinking water can cause health complications. While its presence in drinking water is controversial, I am a big fan of topical fluoride, i.e., fluoride that you apply directly to your teeth via either a fluoride treatment that you receive at the dental office or in a special high-fluoride toothpaste. Since it is topically applied, it goes directly to the area that needs it and does not circulate as widely through your whole system.

You may remember being asked to swish a fluid around in your mouth for a full minute the last time you were at the dentist; that is one way to get fluoride directly to your teeth. There are a couple of problems with this method though. First, no one can actually swish vigorously for a full minute: our cheeks get too tired, and as a result the fluoride doesn't get as well distributed as it should. Then, once we spit, that's it—the fluoride is gone. It is no longer on our teeth, which is where it needs to be.

For these reasons, I prefer applying fluoride as a varnish by literally painting it onto the teeth, where it hardens. It does eventually dissipate, but it sticks around for a matter of hours, as opposed to the thirty seconds or one minute we get with the fluid. The whole goal of fluoride is to get it on our teeth frequently and for as long as possible each time. In fact, toothpaste is more effective if you don't rinse after you spit it out. Spit out the excess, but don't then take a big glug of water and swish it around. Again, the whole idea is to try to get the fluoride to sit on our teeth for a longer period of time, as well as more frequently, which is why it's important to brush at least a couple of times a day.

However, if you are suffering from serious tooth sensitivity, toothpaste really just puts a Band-Aid over a problem with an underlying cause. Tooth sensitivity, or the exposure of the pores of the teeth, is always caused by something else, and, in order to really address sensitivity, we need to know what that is. Here I discuss the two main reasons.

The first one is a relatively easy fix. Many foods and beverages are highly acidic, and that acid wears away enamel (the hard shell on the outside of your teeth), exposing the pores underneath. That's just one of the reasons that drinking soda is so bad for people. All sodas—in fact, the vast majority of products that you get out of a bottle (even many bottled waters)—are acidic enough to dissolve enamel and cause tooth erosion. If you are in the habit of having a Coke or Mountain Dew nearby that you sip on over the course of a day, like our friend Nate from the beginning of the chapter, then your teeth are sitting in a nice little acid bath all day. Every time the pH level in your mouth gets back down to a normal level, you take another sip. Prolonged exposure to that acidity greatly speeds up the breakdown of the enamel. The faster the enamel goes away, again, the more the pores are exposed and the more sensitive the teeth become.

> **If you are in the habit of having a Coke or Mountain Dew nearby that you sip on over the course of a day, like our friend Nate from the beginning of the chapter, then your teeth are sitting in a nice little acid bath all day.**

Citric acid also causes this erosion. If it sits on our teeth, eventually it will dissolve the outer coating. If you snack on oranges, try rinsing with a glass of water after you finish. This will flush the acid off your teeth. (It is not recommended that you brush your teeth immediately after eating citrus or having some other acid on your teeth. Because of the acid, the tooth may be in a compromised state so that brushing could actually contribute to the loss of enamel.)

The erosion of enamel also allows bacteria to more easily create cavities. At the end of the day, cavities—which just result from the accumulation of bacteria in the pores of your teeth—are largely a function of modern diet, a Western modernized problem. So the fix here is straightforward (if not easy): just stop consuming things that eat away at your teeth, or consistently rinse acidic materials off of your teeth after you consume them.

However, there is another common cause of sensitivity that is not so straightforward or easy to fix: clenching and grinding your teeth when you sleep. This is another condition that affects about one in three people, and many don't even know they do it. This can cause cracks in the enamel or even break off small pieces of it, exposing the pores in our teeth.

Clenching and grinding has other effects that can be signs that you have a problem with this sleep habit. Most obvious are chips or cracks on the front teeth or problems with fillings or crowns that break repeatedly. Clenchers and grinders may also experience frequent headaches, migraines, or neck pain due to overworking the muscles of their jaws.

The most common treatment for sensitivity due to clenching and grinding is the night guard, a clear plastic tray that goes over the teeth while you sleep. While it's not terribly attractive, it goes a long way toward creating an environment for tooth sensitivity to disappear. While you may still clench and grind, the damage is done to the plastic of the guard rather than your teeth. The body has repair mechanisms that will take it from there. The problem with clenching and grinding is that you are damaging your teeth at a rate faster than the body is able to repair the area. The night guard basically gives the body a chance to catch up.

This is why, while toothpaste can certainly play a role in the fight against tooth sensitivity, the problem will only get worse, and more difficult to fix, if the root problem is not addressed—whether that root problem be diet, clenching and grinding, or (as is often the case) a combination of the two. The toothpastes should be used in conjunction with healing, not hiding, the cause of tooth sensitivity.

DAMAGE CONTROL

In some cases, either because of breakage or because of the accumulation of bacteria, a tooth will be damaged beyond what the body can naturally repair. This brings us to the topic of fillings and crowns. As I mentioned, cavities result from the accumulation of bacteria in the pores of the teeth. This often results in a pinpoint hole in the tooth, especially between teeth or right along the gum line. This is when the type of fillings that most people are familiar with are appropriate.

A filling involves the rather simple procedure of cutting a little slot in the tooth with a drill (cutting away the decayed or diseased part and leaving as much healthy tooth structure as possible) and filling it with some kind of filling material. Dentists don't always agree on what kind of material is best for this purpose.

Traditional black mercury restoration (filling), also known as amalgam, was first introduced to dentistry in 1819. It has been the tried-and-true dental filling for nearly two hundred years. First things first: black mercury fillings work, and they will last for a long time. They are also the cheapest way to fix a tooth. Very few dentists will argue with any of these statements.

However, the other point of view is that there are potential downsides. What are those? Well, the name says it all: "black mercury." First, these fillings are black, which is (hopefully) not the color of the teeth that they are going into. This is the aesthetic downside.

As for the "mercury": the metal mercury is, in fact, the predominant material in this type of filling. Now, the science shows that once the material is hardened, the toxic mercury is no longer active. However, when you eat, chew gum, or salivate, some mercury vapor does escape. The FDA has decided what is an acceptable amount of mercury exposure for an American. According to them, even if every tooth in your mouth has a mercury filling, you are under that amount. So, they say, you can rest assured that they are healthy.

However, the FDA also came out with a ruling recently that said all dental offices in the United States must have mercury amalgam separators to ensure that no mercury gets into the water supply and back to the general population. Furthermore, in order to dispose of any mercury that is not actually going into a patient's mouth, a practice has to invite a hazmat team to carry it away under lock and key. This raises issues for people who are concerned about what they are putting in their mouths—especially when it will stay there for decades.

Other problems with black mercury fillings are just the result of having a piece of metal in your mouth. As the metal corrodes, it seals increasingly to the tooth; in other words, it works best when it corrodes. In the meantime, like any metal, the filling can expand or contract as it is exposed to hot and cold, and the expansion can sometimes be extreme enough that it starts substantially pushing out against the rest of the tooth. This leads to a greatly increased risk of fractures forming in the tooth. Finally, the metal in the filling also obstructs X-ray imaging of the tooth; because of this, decay can develop underneath the fillings and be difficult or impossible for a dentist to see. In fact, in my experience, I have discovered hidden decay in about half of the cases that involve removing old mercury amalgam fillings.

Many dentists consider black mercury fillings antiquated for all of these reasons, though many dentists also still use them as the easiest and most affordable option. I fall more into the first camp, mainly due to the fact that I know there is now better technology available to repair teeth. I am very careful about what I am willing to put in my patients' mouths, so I have opted to do fillings with a tooth-colored plastic; not only is it more aesthetically pleasing but it functions just as well without raising the concerns about mercury fillings.

CUTTING-EDGE CROWNS AND CERAMICS

When damage or decay goes beyond these small holes, either wrapping around the tooth or being on the chewing surface, a dental crown becomes the better option. Traditionally, a dental crown has completely covered the tooth on all sides and, thus, demanded the removal of a good deal of tooth all around. This type of full crown does not discriminate between good and bad material (remember, with a filling we remove the bad and leave as much good as possible); everything must go. So it is very destructive to the tooth.

Sometimes a full crown is necessary—namely, when a tooth is so badly broken down that it has to be covered with something else that just looks like a tooth. Again, however, new technology makes it possible to avoid this in most cases. My practice has invested in cutting-edge technology that can not only place a crown in one day but can place either a full or a *partial* crown.

A partial crown fits like a puzzle piece into an opening made in the already-existing tooth. To make this opening, we remove the bad while leaving as much of the good tooth as possible. In other words, we remove much less of the original tooth than we would for a full crown. The tooth maintains its structure, which can mitigate problems down the road—typically, the more tooth you're able to save, the fewer problems you will have with that tooth later on.

The CEREC ("ceramic reconstruction") is a CAD/CAM machine, meaning it employs computer-aided design and manufacturing, that designs the crown by taking 3-D pictures of the area in need of repair and constructing a 3-D image of the crown. Powder is applied to the tooth to create a reflective surface, a camera is used to capture the shape of the tooth in 3-D, and the crown is designed on a computer screen directly in front of the patient. That is how the information is obtained, instead of taking an impression of the patient's teeth.

The CEREC then sends that information to the in-office milling unit to actually create the crown. This unit features dental drills surrounding a block of ceramic, which is held in place while the dental drills carve out a crown in the shape of the 3-D image constructed by the CEREC. We then bond the ceramic crown to the tooth. Unlike cement, which is less stable, the bonding material uses the millions of tiny pores in the tooth to almost fuse tooth and crown together, making it stay on and protect the tooth more effectively. This solidifies the structure of the tooth as a whole, making it stronger than it was the day it came into the patient's mouth.

So the CEREC helps us strengthen the tooth and has the added advantage of allowing us to design, create, and place the crown all in a single visit. This is good for the patient, who gets to avoid coming in for a second appointment, and good for the tooth—the sooner we repair the damage, the better.

Only about one in sixteen dentists have made the investment in this technology, which means that the far more common method of placing a crown starts with the messy molds or impressions on the patient's teeth, which no one likes and which are not as accurate as 3-D imaging technology. The patient then wears a temporary, which is vulnerable to bacteria and sensitivity, for a couple of weeks while the crown is created. Then the patient faces the real possibility that the crown will not fit or stay on once it is placed—since, again, impressions aren't as accurate as 3-D imaging. It is common for people to go into their appointment to get their crown seated or fitted, and it doesn't fit or doesn't completely seal the tooth. In these cases, they have to do everything over again, get a temporary back on, and come back for another appointment down the road. (Just look up David Letterman's routine about dealing with the process of getting a crown to see how ridiculous the process can be.)

The CEREC allows us to avoid all of this: the impressions, the temporary crown, the wait for the second appointment, and the frustration of having to go through it all again. Speaking as a dentist, I know that the partial crown from the CEREC would definitely be my preference for repairing any damage to my own teeth. Patients tend to prefer it as well: I had one patient get positively excited when I told her about the CEREC process. She had already had several crowns and was dreading the process until I told her that, among other things, we would not have to take impressions.

She looked at me wide-eyed and said, "No goop?" I just nodded and replied, "No goop—and only one visit." Dentists don't get to hear their patients cheer all that often; this was an exception.

I was thrilled to be able to make the process so much easier and less painless for her; but I also emphasized that the technology allowed me to better serve her from the standpoint of her overall health as well. While treatments like crowns may seem to take us into the world of cosmetic dentistry, I always want to emphasize that dental health plays a role in overall bodily health.

With my own patients, I work hard to attend to and be aware of the impact of their dental health, and how I am affecting it, on their overall health. Surprisingly, in some cases, your dentist may be able to point out to you potential health risks that you are up against; he or she may even be the one who can best help you overcome a health problem, even if that problem doesn't seem to directly have anything to do with your teeth. One clear example of this is sleep apnea, which I discuss in the next chapter.

CHAPTER 3

MORE THAN A SNORE: SLEEP APNEA

"I was banished to the guest room years ago. My snoring would keep my wife up through the night, and while she was awake, she would be waiting and listening for me to take a breath. As a romantic, I knew just what to do when Valentine's Day came around last year: I went to my doctor, who sent me to a sleep specialist, who then diagnosed me with sleep apnea.

"To treat it he prescribed the CPAP. Now I wear an octopus mask that roars like a jet engine all night. I stopped snoring, but my wife wasn't interested in sleeping beside Darth Vader, so I'm back in the guest room. Can you save my marriage—or at least get me out of the guest room?"

This sounds like a tall order for a dentist, but I've heard this type of story many times; and, in fact, I was able to help this gentleman, with the help of a small, silent, portable mouthpiece. Many people don't realize that sleep apnea is a medical condition that their dentist can help with. Worse, many people don't realize how serious sleep apnea is and how important it is to get it treated. This is a major way in which dentistry can powerfully contribute to a person's overall health.

WANT TO LEARN MORE ABOUT THE ELITE SMILE EXPERIENCE? CHAPTER 3 COVERS:

- **what is sleep apnea?**
  - sleep apnea definition
  - negative effects of sleep apnea
- **upper airway resistance syndrome**
- **who is affected?**
  - sleep apnea and sleep breathing disorders in children
  - sleep apnea diagnosis
- **sleep apnea treatments**
  - CPAP
  - OAT

WHAT IS SLEEP APNEA?

Obstructive sleep apnea, as important a problem as it is, has long been un- or underdiagnosed. This is partly because it is a relatively newly discovered problem. It was first diagnosed in the 1960s, and diagnoses have increased over the years. In the last five to ten years especially, the number of diagnoses of sleep apnea has skyrocketed.

I think the recent uptick in diagnoses is due to two factors, the first being simply increasing awareness of sleep apnea. Second, there is a correlation between sleep apnea and obesity; obesity rates are also increasing, and people in our population are gaining weight on average.

Obesity is not the cause of sleep apnea though—I have certainly had fit and trim people walk through the door of my practice who have had severe sleep apnea. This is because it is also partly a matter of genetics. Just as we all have different facial features due to our genetic makeup, we have different internal features as well. In the case of sleep apnea, someone's tongue could be differently shaped or attached in a way that increases the likelihood of sleep apnea.

When adults sleep, their jaws tend to fall backward, taking the tongue with it. Sleep apnea occurs when the tongue has a tendency to fall backward and block the airway, preventing the person from breathing. An "apneic event" occurs when this obstruction prevents the person from taking a breath for four seconds or more. Essentially, the sleeper is going through moments during the night when he or she is literally suffocating for a short period of time. The lungs are trying to take in air, but the airway is completely blocked. Typically, the sleeper will wake slightly and take a gasp of air or will snore loudly as the air forces its way through.

In the meantime, though, the sleeper is literally suffocating. This causes the amount of oxygen in the blood (the blood oxygen saturation level) to decrease, which can have dramatic effects.

When someone is put under general anesthesia for surgery, one of the attendants in the room will be monitoring his or her blood oxygen saturation level, which is expressed as a percentage. If the patient's numbers drop to around 93 or 92 percent, it becomes a concern, and the doctors and attendants have to intervene to bring that level back up. Keep that in mind when I tell you: some apneics' blood oxygen saturation can get as low as *the low eighties or even high seventies* during an apneic event. If these levels were reached in an OR, attendants would be alarmed that they were dealing with a dying patient. During a severe apneic event, the sleeper is actually dying for a few moments—so he or she should really get that checked out.

The decrease in the overall level of oxygen in the blood can also be linked to a number of medical conditions. It can increase your risks of having a heart attack, stroke, and diabetes. It increases your cholesterol, your blood pressure, and the amount of weight you gain. Many doctors won't bother to treat what they consider mild sleep apnea; but if your doctor tells you that you have this and yet doesn't seem concerned, take it with a grain of salt. Mild sleep apnea, unchecked, will eventually turn into moderate sleep apnea, which, unchecked, will eventually turn into severe sleep apnea.

Also, even mild apnea is disturbing to your sleep, which is a basic human need. Most apneics never get into deep REM sleep, which is really our brain's way of resting from the amount of work that it has to do. The light sleep of the apneic won't do the trick. We need the deep levels to help our brains basically clean out the garbage from the day. Without that, we just can't think as clearly; ultimately, we can't be who we are or who we want to be. Having our sleep constantly interrupted prevents us from being able to do so.

Also, the gasping that occurs in sleep apnea is very irritating, not just to your sleeping partner but also to the tissue in your airway, so it leads to inflammation throughout your airway. Walking around with a swollen airway all the time has two major effects: it increases the likelihood of another apneic moment, and it increases the amount of C-reactive protein in the body, with all of the negative health effects we discussed in the previous chapter.

Finally, the blockage of the airway leads the sleeper to instinctively clench and grind his or her teeth—again, along with all of the negative effects we discussed before.

THE SPECTRUM OF DISORDER

Many people can actually have many of the same negative reactions from a similar sleep breathing disorder called upper airway resistance syndrome (UARS). UARS, while not as severe as sleep apnea, can still be very harmful. Interestingly, it often affects young women who are very thin and petite. For example, I was contacted by a woman named Debra who lived in Colorado but had family in my area. In fact, her father had been a patient of mine, and I had helped him with his sleep apnea. This is why she had called me: her local doctors insisted that she didn't have sleep apnea, but she was desperate for someone to help her.

The problem was that she could not sleep more than an hour at a time, even though she was continually exhausted and fatigued. Her lack of sleep was having a severely detrimental effect on her quality of life, causing debilitating migraines on a regular basis (more than once a week). She was starting to miss more and more work, and she had to sleep on a makeshift bed she set up in her closet because she needed complete darkness to recover.

Her doctors had been unable to find the source of the problem, so, after corresponding with her online, I suggested she fly out to come see us. When she arrived, I realized that her appearance was consistent with that of other patients I had seen with UARS: she was short and thin, even frail. Her teeth were in fairly good shape but showed clear signs of grinding. This struck me as a clear case of UARS.

UARS causes a narrowing of the airway that restricts the amount of oxygen you get while sleeping, causing you to be unable to fall into a deep REM sleep. Like sleep apnea, it doesn't necessarily make you fully wake up, but it does prevent your brain from being able to do the cleansing work that gets done in deep sleep, which makes waking life much more difficult—this is why sleep deprivation is a form of torture.

Fortunately, UARS can be treated in much the same way as sleep apnea. In fact, for Debra, I prescribed the same oral device that I had given to her father, and the results were immediate. She slept five hours the first night she used it, and her amount of REM sleep increased night after night from there. She was getting a full night's sleep within a couple of weeks, and her migraines disappeared altogether over the course of a few months—no more missing work or missing out on life.

WHO IS AFFECTED?

Like other problems related to dentistry, sleep apnea and other sleep breathing disorders may not seem like a big deal immediately, but they contribute to a vicious cycle that can end up having extreme negative effects. We need to be able to sleep not just to clear our minds but for the body to be able to repair itself properly. The increase in diagnoses of sleep apnea goes along with trends toward people getting less and less sleep due to technology or having too much to do, and thus not getting the quality of sleep that they need. One of the most disturbing trends is the failure to recognize sleep breathing disorders like apnea in children and babies, which also can have severe effects.

Most cases of ADHD can be linked to sleep breathing disorders.[1] Many kids who suffer from these are not getting enough sleep and have never gotten a good night's sleep in their lives. They lose quality sleep and are not getting the oxygen that they need at night; then they act out, they lose interest in things, they have trouble in

---

1   Shur-Fen Gau S., "Prevalence of sleep problems and their association with inattention/hyperactivity among children aged 6-15 in Taiwan," *Journal of Sleep Research* 19, no. 2 (June 2010): 379, https://www.ncbi.nlm.nih.gov/pubmed/17118097.

school—all the symptoms of something like ADHD; and it can be traced back to sleep. You would probably have behavior problems too if you got a bad night's sleep every night.

Diagnosing a child with ADHD and medicating him or her only treats the symptom of an underlying problem. If the kid could get some relief, and just get a solid night's sleep, his or her problem could be addressed. The oral appliance therapy (OAT) that I discuss would help (if you can get your kid to wear it at night), but most likely his or her tonsils and adenoids are inflamed, and we want to get that inflammation out of the body. In that case, the removal of the tonsils and adenoids can bring relief.

It is worth noting that diagnoses of ADHD continue to go up and up, while, during this same time frame, the number of doctors willing to do surgery to remove a child's tonsils and adenoids has gone down. This surgical procedure may have been common when you were young; I grew up knowing plenty of kids who had had their tonsils removed. Tonsillectomies reached a peak level in the seventies and have been steadily declining since then (mainly because of falling insurance reimbursements), so now it is far from the routine measure it once was.

Dentists and orthodontists, however, are increasingly recommending tonsillectomies prior to getting braces, since the tonsils have a drastic effect on the airway, and this can in turn affect jaw formation and the placement of the teeth. At the same time that we were seeing tonsillectomies decrease, however, we also witnessed a drastic rise in the diagnoses of ADHD, which is treated with medication. ADHD, though, is only the symptom of the problem, which is allowed to continue to affect the child.

Sleep breathing disorders affect kids in other ways too. For instance, kids who continue to wet the bed regularly for years after they should have outgrown this behavior could likely have a sleep breathing problem. These disorders can also cause snoring in children, which should not be occurring. If your child snores regularly—not just when he or she has dozed off in the car seat with his or her neck kind of crooked but on a regular basis, at night, in bed—that is a sleep breathing problem. Finally, and most tragically, sleep breathing problems of some sort are involved in virtually every case of sudden infant death syndrome (SIDS).

When it comes to adults, sleep breathing disorders like sleep apnea, UARS, or even milder snoring (what is known as "primary snoring") are often more immediately distressing for the person sleeping with the sufferer than for the sufferer himself or herself (and, yes, women can suffer from apnea as well as men). Partners are often kept awake by the sound of snoring, which is the sound of air getting past some obstacle that is blocking or constricting the airway. Snoring itself is not a sign of sleep apnea—many people experience simple snoring with no adverse health effects. Also (and more surprisingly for a lot of people), many apneics do not snore at all; their apnea is so severe that their airway is completely blocked, so no air can get by to produce the sound, and they periodically gasp for air as I described earlier—which, again, can be very disturbing to their sleeping partners.

For this reason, diagnosis of sleep apnea often occurs at the request, encouragement, or command of a spouse or partner. The apneic himself or herself might have no idea it is a problem—all of this happens while they are asleep, after all. (This tends to make treatments a hard sell.)

When someone comes to my practice for a sleep apnea diagnosis, we start with a sleep test. We actually provide a monitor that the patient can take home to run the test there. Most people are familiar with the type of sleep test where you have to go to a sleep lab and get hooked up to a bunch of wires, someone watches you as you sleep, and you're in a clinical type of environment. It's really just an unpleasant experience. With our home test, you are in your own comfortable environment and you can do it on your own time, so it is much more comfortable and convenient. Also, the research indicates that the resulting measurements are, for the most part, equivalent to the sleep lab test.

That test will help us determine whether you only have primary or simple snoring, or if it is something more sinister, such as obstructive sleep apnea. If it is the latter, we highly recommend treatment of some sort—again, sleep apnea has major health implications. In fact, treatment could very well add a decade to an apneic's life (or, to look at it from a different direction, untreated sleep apnea can cut a decade off a person's life—which, sadly, I have seen happen). Fortunately, it is becoming significantly easier to treat it.

THE RIGHT CHOICE

There are two prominent treatment options for sleep apnea. The first is the well-known CPAP (continuous positive airway pressure) machine, which the medical community tends to prefer and which insurance companies are typically willing to pay for. With the CPAP, the patient wears a mask that covers his or her face, and the machine pumps air through that mask into the airway. Essentially, it forces air past the obstruction through brute force; the air comes at the blockage so powerfully that it basically shoulders its way past and heads down the windpipe.

The CPAP absolutely works to assure that the sleeper gets air and does not lose oxygen. However, it has a number of downsides.

First, it is very uncomfortable, and many patients can't stand sleeping with it. It is also loud enough that it disturbs the apneic's sleeping partner almost as much as the apnea itself does (hence the complaints of the wife of the gentleman from the beginning of this chapter). For those who need to travel, the size of the CPAP makes it prohibitively difficult to take with them away from home. For all of these reasons, it has a fairly low compliance rate—that is, only about 20 percent of the people who are prescribed the CPAP actually use it regularly and properly. As I said, the CPAP works, but it only works if the mask is actually on your face and the machine is turned on when you sleep.

Even when it is used, though, it simply goes around the airway's blockage rather than actually preventing the blockage from occurring. In a sense, then, it leaves the problem in place and just works around it. In fact, the area can become further inflamed because of the jet engine's worth of air being forced through it. This inflammation only makes the obstruction, and thus the apnea, worse if the CPAP is not used continuously. So the CPAP can actually inadvertently exacerbate the problem. Finally, the clenching and grinding of teeth that occurs alongside sleep apnea will typically still occur with the CPAP.

For all of these reasons, many patients prefer, and the American Academy of Sleep Medicine (which includes dentists) recommends, what is known as "oral appliance therapy" (OAT), also sometimes called a "mandibular advancement device" or MAD. The OAT is a mouthpiece that actually prevents the obstruction from happening. The one I prescribe is the SomnoMed, which prevents the jaw from falling backward while the patient sleeps. By preventing this, the device also keeps the tongue forward; the root structure of the tongue—which is the portion that tends to collapse and fold back on itself, closing off the airway—thus stays in place.

The OAT thus prevents the problem from occurring; the muscle that would form the obstruction in the airway ends up staying out of the way. The OAT also prevents the clenching and grinding that goes along with sleep apnea. If the sleeper is a clencher and grinder independently of his or her sleep apnea, the mouthpiece will still play a protective role like a night guard. Any inflammation in the throat will be alleviated by the OAT, leaving the body in a position to repair itself more effectively.

It is not as uncomfortable as the CPAP, it is silent, and it is small and portable for easy travel. For all of these reasons, its compliance rate is almost exactly the inverse of the CPAP's: whereas only 20 percent of patients who are prescribed the CPAP actually use it, almost 80 percent of those who are prescribed the OAT use it.

OAT will treat simple snoring also, however, we do not typically prescribe it unless the patient has full-on apnea, because we can treat simple snoring with the less elaborate and expensive snore guard. The snore guard, while not rigid or strong enough to hold the jaw fully forward to treat sleep apnea, does the trick just fine for snoring.

In spite of all this, the CPAP remains the predominant method for treating sleep apnea. Why is this? Well, as you may have guessed, the answer comes down to cost. As I mentioned, medical doctors tend to prefer prescribing the CPAP for two reasons. First, medical insurance will more willingly reimburse for the expense of the CPAP, while insurance companies are a little more reluctant to help pay for an OAT. The payment for the CPAP is a relatively straightforward process. Second, though along the same lines, the medical doctor can certainly *prescribe* the OAT device, but he or she cannot actually *make* it. Since it has to be customized to fit the patient's mouth, it has to be created by a dentist. Thus, it is covered, if at all, by different insurance.

Still, for patients with sleep apnea, the cost is typically worth it. Like I said, it could add a decade to their lives, and I have, sadly, seen patients neglect treatment due to the cost and pass away at a much younger age than they would have if they had been treated. Yes, the CPAP is more affordable; but it has all of the drawbacks mentioned previously. Besides, it isn't worth anything if you don't actually use it, which is statistically likely.

GETTING PERSONAL

It may seem strange to see a book about dentistry devote a whole chapter to a sleep disorder. This just illustrates one of the key themes of the book: oral and dental health is a key part of, and is deeply interconnected with, other aspects of overall health. It might not occur to many people to talk to their dentist about sleep problems, so it might surprise them how much insight a dentist can offer. Successful treatment of sleep apnea, a condition with severe medical implications, involves dental knowledge.

Dentistry is part of the project of holistic self-care. Dental care contributes to overall health, and neglecting it can have severe negative effects on physical health down the line. It can even have major effects on a person's mental health or psychological well-being, as we will see in the following chapters. Many people don't realize the seriousness of even what is considered "cosmetic" dentistry, but it is a major part of my practice because I see self-confidence and a healthy smile as part of one's overall wellness.

PART II

DENTISTRY AND CONFIDENCE: THE SMILE MAKEOVER

CHAPTER 4

NO MORE MISSING TEETH: IMPLANTS

t has happened to me before, but it is always jarring: a patient bursts
into tears as soon as I walk into the room. Some are terrified of
dentists. Some of them are so overwhelmed with the problems they
are having with their teeth that they don't know what to do anymore.

One patient, let's call her Liz, was both. "I've always been afraid
of dentists," she told me, "so much so that I've been walking around
with this partial denture that broke years ago. It fits poorly; it's just
ugly. I'm embarrassed to smile, but I was so afraid to see you that I
just put up with it until now."

I handed Liz a tissue and a bottle of water and got to work—by
which I mean I sat down and had a conversation with her. By the end
of it she was at ease and had an understanding of how I might be able
to help her. I looked in her mouth then and saw that she would need
nine implants in various spots around her mouth. Over the course of
the next few months, we did the implants and watched them heal.
She was petrified at the beginning of every visit but grateful by the

end of the process. "I can eat and laugh like I did when I was much younger, and I can smile again," she told me.

That last remark just goes to show the profound impact that cosmetic dentistry can have on a person's life. Eating, laughing, and smiling are not just matters of vanity; they are central aspects of our lives and of our psychological well-being.

WANT TO LEARN MORE ABOUT THE ELITE SMILE EXPERIENCE? CHAPTER 4 COVERS:

- **the significance of cosmetic dentistry**
  - bullying
  - self-confidence and our smiles

- **replacing teeth**
  - the development of the dental implant
  - the importance of replacing your teeth

- **how does it work?**
  - parts of a dental implant
  - the process of getting an implant

- **what does an implant accomplish?**
  - effects of losing molars
  - effects of losing front teeth

- **treatments for multiple missing teeth**
  - traditional dentures (and why everyone hates them)
  - snap dentures
  - all-on four technology

THE SIGNIFICANCE OF COSMETIC DENTISTRY

With the rise of social media, bullying has taken center stage as an issue in recent years. It is a problem many people—adults as well as children—face. It is not isolated to the schoolyard but can occur in the workplace as well. Just as it is damaging for kids, it can take a serious emotional toll on adults as well, leading to decreased productivity at work or even avoiding the workplace altogether. It is a prevalent problem that we are all susceptible to, whether we are getting bullied or a loved one is.

Why are people bullied? I can't comment on the psychology of bullies, but the American Academy of Orthodontists (AAO) recently completed a study that showed the number-one target of bullying is a person's smile. Children also report that comments about their teeth were among the most hurtful types of bullying; and just imagine the harmful psychological effects of essentially being discouraged from smiling day after day.

The purpose of the AAO study was to look at how bullying affected self-esteem, school performance, and school attendance; kids who suffer from this type of bullying are much more likely to struggle academically and miss school. The AAO focuses on braces and the position of your teeth, which affects not only your smile but also your facial features and airway. The AAO found that the four most common dental-facial features that were a target of bullying were spaces between teeth, missing teeth, the shape or color of teeth, and prominent front teeth (often called "buck teeth").

It is important to note that bullying is never the fault of the victim, and no one deserves to be bullied, as none of us is perfect or without flaws. Still, if you were able to change the feature that draws the most attention from bullies, wouldn't you want to? Many people go through their whole lives being bullied because of their smile. I have had several patients tell me that they had come to me because they just decided, "Enough is enough! I'm going to do this for myself."

Making over a smile can have a significant impact on a person's life. Generally, as many studies have shown, an attractive smile is very important to a person's self-confidence, and improving one's smile can lead to improvements in mental health or psychological well-being. It also affects how they are seen by other people. For better or for worse, when someone meets you for the first time, the first thing he or she notices is your smile. The smile is what first impressions are built on, whether it is the schoolyard, a first date, or a job interview. Not only is a smile a *sign* of confidence but if you are confident in your smile, it can be a *source* of confidence as well.

Also, the number-one thing that most people say they would change about their physical appearance is their smile. In our image-conscious, selfie-focused culture, it makes sense that the smile is the thing about ourselves that we are most drawn to. If someone could improve it, simultaneously reducing his or her chances of being bullied and improving the gut reaction people have when they meet him or her—how could this not go a long way toward improving confidence and psychological well-being?

Cosmetic dentistry makes this possible and has implications for overall health as well. For instance, research has recently shown a link between having missing teeth and increased likelihood of dementia. Implants, which I talk about in this chapter, serve to mitigate that risk. Cosmetic dental procedures like implants also affect overall mouth health (and thus, indirectly, overall body health) and the shape of the mouth and airway. We should not underestimate the broader significance of these types of procedures.

REPLACING TEETH

As I just mentioned, the more teeth you are missing, the more likely you are to develop dementia over time. We can add that to the more obvious problems with missing teeth, such as having a more difficult time chewing your food or being embarrassed to smile or talk. Having teeth missing also makes you more prone to frequent headaches and even migraines. More importantly, it can transform the health of your mouth, putting you at higher risk of decay and gum disease. Surrounding teeth may start to move in to try to refill the space where a tooth is missing, which can alter your bite and cause jaw pain. Externally, not having some or all of your teeth in place may cause your mouth to shrink in, making you look—and feel—older than you actually are.

For thousands of years now, people have recognized and tried to solve these problems associated with losing teeth. Attempts to replace teeth with some kind of substitute go back at least to the ancient Egyptians. The progress made over the centuries has finally brought us the modern-day dental implant, which looks and feels just like a tooth and is the best way to replace a missing tooth.

By around the 1960s or 1970s, the period of experimentation was over and dentists were able to place quality implants with fairly good predictability, so since then we have been able to refine and perfect the process over time. Originally the thinking was that the portion of the implant that went into the jawbone (the anchor) needed to be quite long and thick to be stable. These were basically big old screws that were fifteen millimeters long and five millimeters in diameter. That may not sound like much, but at the end the day, this screw is going into a jawbone, which isn't all that thick; and the screw needs to be completely encased in surrounding bone in order to properly set. Still, the dental community slowly began to realize that smaller, narrower implants would do the trick. We can now do them as short as eight millimeters, even shorter in some cases; and we're routinely placing screws that are three or four millimeters wide.

The size of implants, then, has dropped dramatically; as a result, the number of people who are able to be treated with implants has skyrocketed for the simple reason that patients just don't need to have as much bone in their jaws as we used to think they did in order to get an implant. Implants have also been around long enough, and the science has improved enough, that they are no longer experimental, so the amount of research required to get an implant to market has been significantly reduced, with the result that they are much more affordable than they used to be.

All in all, implants are more accessible and successful than they have ever been, and the number of patients we are able to treat in this way has exploded. My practice has 3-D imaging technology that can allow us to place implants even in patients who may have been told they weren't candidates for implants in the past.

The installation of the implant is a form of surgery, and dentists like to present an air of wonder and mystery around implants. When it comes right down to it, though, there is really nothing magical about them; the mechanism is quite straightforward. It's a great work of medical technology and an amazing treatment to be able to provide. As long as the dentist does everything properly, though, what we really have to thank is the body's ability to accept foreign material and heal itself. The anchor is made of surgical-grade titanium, which is a material the body doesn't reject; it is placed in the bone, and the bone just grows around it.

HOW DOES IT WORK?

The implant itself consists of three parts:

1. Implant/Anchor
2. Abutment
3. Crown

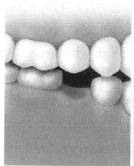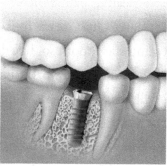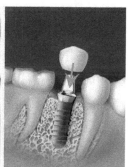

We have already talked about the anchor, a titanium screw that is placed down in the bone to serve as an artificial root. It takes up minimal space and remains sturdy, so you do not feel like something is floating or flopping around in your mouth. As long as the area is not contaminated, the bone will naturally heal around and adhere to the anchor. The anchor is hollow so that something can be placed inside it, and once it is healed, an abutment or post is tightened into it. The post is used to support a dental crown, which feels and looks just like a natural tooth.

The anchor is the key component, and we install it well before the other parts; it only takes about fifteen minutes to install a single anchor, and we use a topical anesthetic, so the procedure is not painful and the patient should be able to go about his or her business after it is over. Ideally, if we are extracting the tooth that we are replacing, we are able to place the implant on the same day that the tooth comes out; this requires the use of grafting material, which is basically sterilized bone tissue that helps the bone grow around the anchor. This method preserves the bone as much as possible and speeds up the healing process.

Typically, we need about three months of healing time for the implant to be completely accepted by the bone. During the time that the bond is bonding to the implant, which we call the "integration period," we can screw a healing cap, which looks like a little silver mushroom, into the implant. Or, if we are replacing a front tooth, we can give the patient a temporary tooth so they don't go without being able to smile at all for those three months. Either the healing cap or the temporary tooth will basically keep the implant itself accessible to us over the course of the healing process.

After that healing period, we run into a step where technology can make all the difference. My practice has invested in technology that allows us to test the healing of the implant without applying any force to it. We basically place a little peg inside of the implant, and then we hold a radio frequency wand (we call it our "magic wand") up to the implant, and it spits out a number. As long as that number is where it needs to be, then the bone has healed as much as it needs to and we're ready to go. We just replace the healing cap with the abutment, and soon we're done with it. Once the crown is in place, it can be used just like a natural tooth.

Most offices don't have this "magic wand" technology; instead, they test the healing process by placing an instrument in the implant and applying a tremendous amount of force to it. If it moves, then it isn't ready. The downside of that is that, if it hasn't healed enough, it moves. If it moves, then it's done for—they have to take the implant out and start the process all over. For that reason, instead of three months, most offices wait closer to six months before testing the implant because they don't want to take a chance on the fact that the implant hasn't had enough time to heal.

In our case, if the implant hasn't had enough time to heal, we just pop the healing cap or temporary back on there and see you in another month. Our significantly less invasive way of testing the implant really speeds up the whole process.

WHAT DOES AN IMPLANT ACCOMPLISH?

This simple three-part mechanism can accomplish a great deal and have a profound effect on a person's life. An implant fully replaces, and can last as long as, a real tooth, as long as it is kept clean; only 5 percent of implants fail, typically due to the presence of bacteria. When we're thinking about tooth loss, it is clear that there are basically two categories of tooth that people can lose: back (i.e. molars) and front. The implant treats both types of tooth loss effectively, but to appreciate the value of the implant, we should look at the different types of effect each type of tooth loss can have.

The molars are our chewing teeth, and we're only given eight of them (twelve if you count wisdom teeth, which people tend to have removed). This means that, if we lose one molar (which people often do), the upper or lower that corresponds to it is now useless. Loss of a molar thus means loss of 25 percent of one's chewing ability or functionality. This decrease in our ability to chew causes the other teeth to work harder.

If you've ever done a group project, you may know how frustrating it is when someone isn't doing their fair share of the work. This may lead to being overworked and/or to acting out in some way. Well, teeth behave the same way. Putting extra stress on our teeth leads them to act out by doing things like chipping, breaking, or becoming more sensitive. This kind of damage might need a crown and could eventually even lead to more tooth loss; and we have the beginning of yet another vicious cycle, because the loss of one tooth has caused the others to be overworked and overstressed.

Loss of a second molar will mean we've now lost 50 percent of our chewing ability, and now we're doing more chewing with our front teeth. The front teeth aren't designed to chew, though; they're designed to bite and cut food and push it to the big guys in the back for chewing. If the front teeth are now doing work that they weren't designed to, they start breaking down as well, and the vicious cycle moves to the front. So, with molars, it really is best to replace those teeth as quickly as possible so that the other teeth don't have to carry the extra burden of being overworked and eventually breaking down themselves.

This leads us to losing teeth in the front, which has more of a cosmetic effect. Apart from biting functionality, though, even the psychological and emotional effect of missing front teeth can be quite significant. Like I said before, a person's smile is a key aspect of his or her self-confidence, and being embarrassed to smile or having to cover your mouth when you smile can have a social impact and affect your mood. Suppressing your smile can even make you more depressed. I have had many patients cry in my chair about their smile—especially those who are missing a tooth in the front. It affects performance at work and in social settings; it is detrimental overall.

Finally, as I mentioned before, losing teeth and not replacing them has been associated with an increased likelihood of dementia. This is a very significant role an implant could potentially play.

TAKING IT FURTHER

If someone has a lot of teeth missing or broken down, implants can also replace entire sets of teeth. In a lot of cases, I deal with patients who have had numerous root canals, implants, crowns, and so forth, and are just sick of dealing with their teeth one by one. They've got so many teeth that are broken down that they are reaching a hopeless point where they don't want to continue to throw good money after bad results.

In the past, this problem has been addressed with dentures, which are notoriously frustrating for those who wear them. Both the top and bottom denture are difficult to deal with, though for slightly different reasons. A top denture goes completely over the roof of your mouth and stays in basically through suction adhesion to the roof of your mouth. So the roof of your mouth is covered in acrylic. As you can imagine, a lot of people don't enjoy the sensation of a sheet of plastic across the roof of their mouth. It affects the way food tastes; it affects their breathing; it makes it more difficult to eat. For people who have a strong gag reflex, having plastic extending all the way to their soft palate is problematic and uncomfortable.

A bottom denture stays in basically thanks to the movement of your lips and your tongue. There is no suction adhesion to the floor of your mouth, because that's where your tongue is. As bad as the top denture sounds, almost everyone who has had a set of dentures will tell you they hate the bottom one more than the top one. I don't even bother with giving people dentures on the bottom; if they need them, I go straight to some sort of multi-tooth implants.

Multi-tooth implants allow us to move to a more permanent solution for serious cases. Unlike dentures, which take up a lot of space in your mouth and make it difficult to eat or speak, dental implants feel natural. There are basically two approaches possible for multi-tooth implants: snap dentures and the fixed dental bridge (which is called "all-on-four" technology).

Snap dentures allow multiple teeth to be snapped onto just a couple of anchors. These feel much more natural and stay in place better than traditional adhesive dentures. The process requires us to place a couple of implants that have little snaps on them, and we make a denture of whatever size is needed—no palate portion necessary for the top—that has corresponding snaps so it can just snap into place. No suction or any other type of adhesive required. Snap dentures chew better, allow the patient to breathe and taste his or her food better, and reduce the likelihood of gagging. On the bottom, the snaps give the teeth a home so they're not completely flipping and flopping around on you like a regular bottom denture.

A patient with snap dentures may notice a little bit of micro-movement or flexing of the dentures. To address this, we have a better option even beyond the snap denture: all-on-four technology allows a dental bridge (i.e. a bunch of crowns connected to each other) to actually be screwed into an implant, such that it cannot be taken out. This is the closest we can get to actually replacing your teeth. The fixed dental bridge makes up the entire row of teeth, top or bottom, which is anchored to just four implants (hence the name), and it will not move.

With this technique, we have essentially replaced an entire set of teeth, with a minimal amount of material, in a way that sets your teeth exactly how they were originally supposed to be. The material is extremely strong, and it is even more aesthetically pleasing than the snap denture. All-on-four is really the pinnacle of what we're able to do for someone who is missing many to all of their teeth.

Some patients worry about the cleanliness of these bridges or getting food caught under them. Cleaning is easy enough with the snap denture; the patient is able to take it in and out. We recommend that the implants get cleaned and that the snaps be replaced every once in a while. The fixed dental bridge, on the other hand, can only be removed by a dentist; however, food will not get caught underneath, and patients can clean them themselves with brushing and regular dental visits just like their original teeth.

Tooth loss is more common than people realize, especially as people get older. Since people are also starting to live longer, it is becoming an issue for more and more people. Implants—the all-on-four bridge being the most impressive variety—offer a reliable, healthy, and aesthetically pleasing solution. For people with missing teeth, implants can help them to smile again, which increases quality of life; and for older folks, implants let them have the same look as when they were young, so they feel more youthful, energetic, and optimistic.

CHAPTER 5

STRAIGHTEN UP

O nly four months: that didn't give us a lot of time. For the previous few months, Maggie had been bouncing from dentist to dentist until finally she landed at our office. With each new visit, she was becoming more and more desperate: her wedding was just months away, and she was embarrassed about how the position of her teeth affected her smile. She had lived with it up to this point, but she didn't like seeing herself in photos, and she couldn't stand the thought of not smiling in her wedding pictures or of having wedding pictures she would be embarrassed to look at and to show people.

Every dentist had told her that she had two options: the quicker but very intrusive one (involving an elaborate series of drilling, root canals, veneers, and crowns) or the less intrusive but much longer term one (involving braces and other traditional orthodontic procedures). The first option would have been very costly and destructive and probably would not have given her the results she wanted; and, of course, the second would not fix things in time for her wedding.

By the time she ended up in our office, her wedding was just over four months away, which put us in a tough situation. Hers was one of the most extreme cases I've ever taken on. Her canines on both top and bottom were far out of place—up near her nose on top and down very low on her gum on the bottom. Still, I agreed to try to help her. Fortunately, these were front teeth rather than molars, and her bite was otherwise fine, so I decided to treat her with Elite Speed Braces, a special type of braces that aim to straighten the teeth in six months. I'll explain how this works later.

The plan had been to treat her with the braces for four months, take them off for the wedding, and then put them back on for the remaining couple of months. However, she was so happy with the result after just four months that she just left the braces off. We saved her a really expensive and destructive process, and even though we approached it aggressively, it was no more painful than traditional orthodontics. We now have a beautiful wedding photo of her in our office, and she happily allows us to use her "before and after" shots to show the dramatic effect that our teeth-straightening techniques can have.

WANT TO LEARN MORE ABOUT THE ELITE SMILE EXPERIENCE? CHAPTER 5 COVERS:

- **traditional orthodontics**
  - how it works
  - braces
- **alternatives to braces**
  - Invisalign
  - Elite Speed Braces

IF YOU PUSH IT, IT WILL MOVE

Orthodontics

It's just physics: if you apply enough force to an object, it will move. Apply this basic principle to teeth, and there you have it: orthodontics. Of course, orthodontists want to help teeth move in a certain way, and they have to use gentle force to avoid damaging the teeth or causing the patient excruciating pain, so there's a little more to it than that. When moving teeth, there is a specific configuration that is healthiest and considered most attractive, where the teeth are straightly aligned in a perfect "U" or horseshoe shape; and the goal of orthodontic work is to force the teeth into that formation.

Whenever a child's adult teeth start coming in, there are a number of variables that affect the location and the angle at which they come in, such as the presence of baby teeth obstructing the normal path or oral habits like thumb sucking. The sum total of these effects is the kid's smile; if a kid has several teeth that are misplaced or out of alignment, this will have an aesthetically displeasing effect. It will also have an effect on his or her airway and chewing ability—so again, a smile is not "merely" a cosmetic issue.

Front teeth, for example, can easily come in at an angle that makes them prominently flared outward, producing the effect that people call "buck teeth." This condition is a prime target of the type of bullying discussed in the previous chapter. Often this effect is self-correcting; as the kid continues to grow, the teeth straighten up. In other cases, however, this will become a permanent part of a person's smile unless some sort of orthodontic intervention takes place.

Braces

This type of intervention can take basically three forms—though, again, all three techniques operate on the same principle of gently forcing the tooth to move from its current position to the desired position. The first technique is the one that people typically think of when they think of orthodontics: the "railroad-track"-like braces that involve metal brackets cemented to the teeth and attached to a wire with small bands. The orthodontist periodically adjusts the wire in the direction of the desired position of the teeth, and the wire starts pulling the teeth slowly in that direction.

These braces, of course, are very noticeable; if you want, you can even draw extra attention to them by jazzing them up with multicolored bands. That approach is all well and good when you're thirteen years old, but, since they are often associated with adolescent kids, these braces give off an appearance in adults as being juvenile. Yet the alignment of the teeth can be changed at any age, and adults are increasingly turning to opportunities to improve their smiles through straightening their teeth. Adults may not want to make themselves look more immature by having these railroad tracks on their teeth. Understandably, adults typically prefer a subtler, less noticeable approach when it comes to straightening their teeth.

> *Adults typically prefer a subtler, less noticeable approach when it comes to straightening their teeth.*

Fortunately, new technologies give adults an alternative to traditional metal brackets. Both of the other techniques for straightening teeth offer the opportunity to straighten your smile discreetly, comfortably, and confidently.

THE ADULT ALTERNATIVES TO BRACES

The two techniques that offer an alternative to braces are Invisalign and Elite Speed Braces. Again, like braces, these straighten the smile by forcing the teeth to move. They tend to be more appropriate for adults, as they tend to result in more cosmetic changes, as opposed to the deep structural changes orthodontists try to effect with braces. We can achieve some functional changes through these straightening methods, improving problems with clenching and grinding or opening up the airway, for instance. However, for the type of radical treatment that adolescents often require, traditional braces remain the appropriate option.

Both Invisalign and Elite Speed Braces work by offering a kind of template of ideal tooth position and rounded jaw shape. The apparatus then pushes the jaw and teeth in the direction of the ideal shape with a gentle force.

Invisalign

Invisalign, the most well-known and popular option for adults hoping to straighten their teeth, applies this force with a series of clear plastic trays ("aligners") that are switched out every two weeks. The trays move and align the teeth so that, by the time the patient is finished with the last tray, his or her teeth end up in the appropriate position. This typically takes eleven months to a year.

The aligners are thin and clear so that they are unobtrusive. For the most part, no one can tell that a patient is wearing them; as the name suggests, they are nearly invisible. They allow the patient to eat as normal, and they are removable for cleaning purposes. If worn all day, every day, and taken out only for brushing, then Invisalign will do a wonderful job of moving teeth without anyone else even knowing that the process is going on.

This approach has a number of advantages. It is the most comfortable of the three options, since the progress is slower and gentler; also, the aligners are simple plastic trays, so the patient doesn't have brackets and wires poking and rubbing up against his or her lips and cheeks. Also, we don't really have to worry too much if a patient loses a tray or throws it away for some reason, because we can just replace it with the next one that's coming without much trouble. It's also more hygienic than traditional orthodontics simply due to the fact that there are no brackets and wires, so the patient can clean his or her teeth more easily. Finally, Invisalign doesn't limit what the patient can eat as much as braces do—there is nothing for chewing gum to get caught up in, and there are no brackets to break off by biting down on something too hard.

Since the trays are removable *and* they are not *completely* invisible, patients will often take them out for an event such as a date or a party, or for photos; this is fine in itself, as long as he or she replaces it as soon as that event is over or the photo is taken. If the treatment is abruptly stopped, the process can start to reverse itself, and the teeth will move back to the old position, which is at that time more natural-feeling for them. One thing I tell patients to keep in mind is that four *hours* without the tray in can cost them four *days'* worth of progress. Taking the aligner out for a special occasion is only a good idea if those special occasions are few and far between. (Friday night is not a special occasion.)

This is actually one of the downsides of Invisalign: too many patients develop the bad habit of taking the aligner out regularly, so they end up losing any of the progress they have been making with the tray in. This also makes it more likely that they will lose trays or leave them at home while they are away. This leads many patients to just give up on Invisalign; they get fed up dealing with the gross, saliva-covered plastic tray that they are constantly putting in and taking out of their mouths. The treatment is also longer and requires more frequent visits to the dentist's office, increasing the odds of burnout.

Still, if a patient is diligent and sticks with the treatment, he or she will see significant effects on the straightness of his or her smile within about a year. The question is just whether the patient is willing to commit to it and keep the treatment up for that whole time period.

While it works more quickly than traditional braces tend to, Invisalign can be seen as the slow and steady option, with the benefits that come with that approach (such as increased comfort), in comparison to Elite Speed Braces. We can also treat more difficult cases with Elite Speed Braces because the changes we can make with it are more drastic. Invisalign is like cleaning a messy house, while Elite Speed Braces is more like a renovation project. For that reason, I tend to treat people who just have minor complaints about tooth placement—one tooth is a bit crooked, or they want to get rid of a gap—with Invisalign. A more thorough smile remodel would be better approached with Elite Speed Braces.

Elite Speed Braces

Elite Speed Braces takes the traditional orthodontics approach to a new level, using brackets and wires to move the teeth like traditional braces, but doing so much more quickly and discreetly. The brackets are made of a tooth-colored nickel titanium; traditional braces have silver-colored brackets. (Sometimes people have the option of clear brackets with traditional braces, but they are still bulky and more noticeable than the tooth-colored Elite Speed Braces brackets.) The wire itself is also coated with a tooth-colored material, so the apparatus as a whole, while still visible, tends to blend in with the surrounding teeth, thus drawing much less attention than traditional braces.

The wire, in this case, is a "U"- or horseshoe-shaped nickel titanium wire that is quite special in that it has an elastic memory. This means that it "remembers" its original shape, so to speak, and it has a tendency to want to return to that shape when it is bent. The original shape of the wire mirrors the desired horseshoe shape of the mouth, so when the wire is bent to align with and be attached to the teeth, it strives to get back to its original shape, taking the patient's whole mouth along with it. It pulls the teeth into the same shape that it wants to achieve, so the teeth end up arranged and positioned in the form of a good-looking smile.

Elite Speed Braces allows us to rapidly move teeth for a dramatic but predictable change in a relatively short period of time. As with traditional braces, there are brackets and wires there, but they are tooth-colored; so Elite Speed Braces is more noticeable than Invisalign but not as much as traditional braces. Also, the patient only has to wear the apparatus for six months, while braces can stay on for years.

Many people are skeptical about the possibility of this kind of change in a short time frame—the kind we were able to achieve with the bride-to-be from the beginning of this chapter—or suspect that it would be very painful. It is important to note here, though, that while Elite Speed Braces operates like traditional braces, it is doing its work for a cosmetic rather than a functional effect, which involves most of the effort of the nickel titanium wire being exerted on the *front* teeth.

The front teeth are considerably easier to move than the molars, which are treated with the type of traditional orthodontics that kids get. Front teeth only have one root, while molars can have two or three. Traditional orthodontics, then, is really a whole different ball of wax: moving one molar requires two to three times the amount of force that moving a front tooth does. This requires a different type of metal, often stainless steel. This metal has no elastic memory, so the orthodontist actually has to shape the wire in such a way that it produces the desired movement. As a result, much more force is applied, which is the cause of the pain from traditional braces.

While in some sense, then, Invisalign and Elite Speed Braces offer an opportunity to pursue a much more aggressive treatment in terms of the change to the way a patient's smile looks, this change is not as structurally intrusive as traditional braces. Neither of these options is any more painful than traditional orthodontics; in fact, while I have had patients complain of the pain that their traditional braces cause, I have never heard this from someone using Invisalign or Elite Speed Braces.

CHANGING COURSE

Traditional orthodontics, of course, has a very important place, especially in treating young people. It should also be kept in mind, though, that some adults will more properly be treated with traditional braces. Many people make it all the way to adulthood with bite problems that can cause jaw pain or even migraines. With a patient who is having these difficulties, it is more appropriate to turn to traditional, comprehensive orthodontics.

For adults simply looking to increase their confidence or the appeal of their smile through straightening and repositioning their teeth, Invisalign and Elite Speed Braces offer different, but equally effective, routes to the desired outcome. One good example is our patient Alice, a deaf woman who grew up being terribly bullied. Her smile was only slightly misaligned in the front and her bite was good, but because kids were already picking on her because of her disability, they piled on her crooked smile as another thing to make fun of.

Because of this, she grew up suppressing her smile, which only made things worse. Finally, at the age of thirty, she decided to do something about it, and we treated her with Invisalign. It made an incredible difference for her smile, for which she is grateful. She always tells us, "You guys always see me smile, but I never smiled before having this done." Her treatment took about nine months, but it will change the course of her life forever.

CHAPTER 6

PERFECTING YOUR SMILE: WHITENING AND VENEERS

nnie from Long Island: that's what she always called herself, and for some reason it stuck in my head. She was a blogger, from Long Island of course, who contacted me via email with some questions about her smile, which she didn't like. We corresponded for a bit, and then I didn't hear from her again ... until a couple of years later, lo and behold! A woman walks into my office and says, "Hey, it's Annie from Long Island; remember me?"

I did remember her. It turns out she was heavily involved in the at-the-time cutting-edge business of retrofitting buildings for LED lightbulbs. She was known for this nationwide, and her notoriety had landed her a spot on a nationally televised home-improvement show. "I'm going to be on TV!" she told me. "That's exciting, but also, I really can't be on TV with my teeth looking like this."

As a kid, she had a bunch of cavities between her teeth and, subsequently, had a bunch of tooth-colored fillings. These fillings were starting to break down, so they were, as dentists put it, "leaking":

the seal that binds the fillings to the teeth had gone bad, allowing bacteria and debris in that could cause staining—especially from red wine and coffee (and Annie from Long Island was a big fan of both). Not only that but the filling material itself was starting to turn a yellowish-brown color. Because of the locations of all these fillings, she always looked like she had stuff stuck between her teeth.

She wanted to make over her smile in preparation for her segment on national TV; this opportunity had come up out of the blue, so she was in a hurry, and this was very important to her. She needed it done quickly, and with veneers and whitening, we were able to get her turned around and her smile made over really quickly, and she was thrilled.

WANT TO LEARN MORE ABOUT THE ELITE SMILE EXPERIENCE? CHAPTER 6 COVERS:

- **the confidence question**
- **whitening**
  - how it works
  - Sinsational Smile
- **dental veneers**

THE CONFIDENCE QUESTION

Annie from Long Island's situation perfectly illustrates the profound effect cosmetic changes to a person's smile can have on his or her personal and psychological well-being. Before her smile makeover, she had found it very hard to smile and was even uncomfortable talking to people face-to-face. This ran the risk of negatively affecting her business, as it made it harder for her to promote and sell her products. The TV show made it urgent, but even before that she had been traveling all over the country to trade shows, doing presentations to potential clients and things like that. Her embarrassment about her smile, even if it wasn't always conscious, had been an obstacle all along the way.

After her smile makeover, on the other hand, things turned around completely. She reported to us that her sales increased almost immediately afterward, and her business grew exponentially in the months that followed. This just confirms the general trend that, for people in marketing positions, their sales improve when they get their smiles redone. Of course, the sales pitch is only one of the many scenarios in which we can benefit from being comfortable smiling. The increased confidence that comes with being able to smile openly and comfortably just improves our personal interactions.

Annie from Long Island started out as a blogger and only slowly became someone who was more in the public eye, doing public speaking. Concealed behind a computer screen, she was able to let her personality, which was very energetic and fun, really come out in a way that she hadn't been comfortable doing in public or face-to-face with others because she just wasn't confident in her smile. Once that confidence increased, she was able to do more public events—and even be on TV.

PEARLIER WHITES

Tooth color is maybe the most basic feature of the teeth that people notice; it's no surprise that there are plenty of products on the shelf designed to whiten teeth, such as special toothpastes and whitening strips. While these can be moderately effective if used consistently over a long period of time, we have dental techniques that can whiten teeth more effectively and more quickly.

All whitening products, whether you find them at the store or at the dentist's office, operate on basically the same principle. As I explained in my discussion of tooth sensitivity, our teeth are covered with microscopic pores, and when these pores are exposed, stuff can get in there. Any time we eat something that would, say, stain a T-shirt, that colorful material gets inside those tiny pores. That coffee or red wine spill on your white shirt has basically the same effect on your teeth when you drink.

Of course, brushing and fluoride treatment are essential to protecting your teeth and keeping them white and clean. However, these stains naturally occur over time, and teeth-whitening technologies have been developed to address this.

The most popular form of whitening involves custom-fit plastic trays that a patient wears at night over the course of a week. These trays contain a gel that is a form of hydrogen peroxide, which gets into the pores and bubbles out all of that gunky material that has clogged the pores over time, returning the patient's teeth more closely to their original, natural white.

The whitening products that can be purchased over the counter contain the same form of hydrogen peroxide, so they work basically on the same principle. However, the bleach comes in a much less concentrated form, so the product requires more consistent repetition of application over a longer period of time. The type prescribed by the dentist has a stronger effect in much less time.

Fastest of all, however, is the method in which dentists use this same gel but expose it to a light that makes the bleach work faster. The light essentially activates the gel, so the patient can just sit exposed to the light for a short period of time in the dentist's office and go home with the same white teeth he or she would have gotten from a week using those little plastic trays. The cutting-edge technology we use in our office, known as "Sinsational Smile," amplifies the effect of the gel so effectively that we can whiten teeth in twenty minutes as opposed to days or weeks. This process involves applying a cleanser that helps to partially open up the pores so that the bleach can dive down deeper and pull out more of that standing material when it's exposed to the light.

> *The cutting-edge technology we use in our office, known as "Sinsational Smile," amplifies the effect of the gel so effectively that we can whiten teeth in twenty minutes as opposed to days or weeks.*

A lot of people hear that the material involved is essentially a form of bleach and it freaks them out—they think it couldn't possibly be healthy. This is not the case; the bleach is not harmful at all. Eating an orange is actually more damaging to your teeth than whitening, due to the citric acid. Also, by removing bacteria from the pores of the teeth, whitening can contribute to overall oral health. And it does not increase the sensitivity of the teeth; while the pores open up, the bleach contains a sensitivity relief formula that mitigates the effect.

This, of course, assumes that the patient has an otherwise healthy mouth. Some studies have shown that, in patients with periodontal disease, whitening can actually increase the red complex bacteria and cause further harm to the gums. So, if you're planning on getting your teeth whitened, make sure you don't have periodontal disease—though, if you have periodontal disease, you really have other things to worry about than getting your teeth whitened.

FINISHING TOUCHES

The dental veneer is the primary tool for the full-on smile makeover. A dental veneer is simply a thin porcelain jacket that slips over the top of a tooth. This type of tooth treatment is considered one of the most versatile cosmetic dentistry procedures because it provides a very natural-looking result. Every veneer is shaped, colored, and sized to perfectly fit the individual who is getting it. They can be bonded to the tooth incredibly quickly and easily, and they are very strong, long-lasting, and resistant to cracking or chipping.

I am a firm believer in dental veneers. I have some myself, as do some of my closest loved ones. Shape, color, and size—basically, anything about a particular tooth that a patient doesn't like—can be addressed with a veneer, for a crisp, natural-looking, white smile. They are the closest thing to a "quick fix" for all kinds of problems with a person's smile. At our office, with advances in technology and highly trained professionals, we can offer a complete smile makeover in a single visit and without giving the patient a single shot or having to take a single impression. Veneers allow us to have complete control over the appearance of a person's smile—so whether the patient wants a literal "Hollywood smile" (and believe me, those celebrity smiles are all achieved with veneers) or just wants to even out the shape and size of his or her teeth, we can achieve that with veneers.

Our teeth really take a beating over time; we chew and bite with them incorrectly, and they can chip and wear in odd ways so that they look malformed. Veneers offer the most straightforward way of addressing this minor wear and tear. In this kind of case, we can do a conservative set of veneers where we don't even touch the actual teeth. We can bond the veneer right to the tooth, so the patient gets a beautiful new smile in a very short period of time.

> *With advances in technology and highly trained professionals, we can offer a complete smile makeover in a single visit and without giving the patient a single shot or having to take a single impression.*

Teeth can also experience sudden trauma—a bicycle accident, for instance—and can actually die in some of these cases. That is, the trauma causes the living tissue inside the tooth to stop functioning and begin to decay. That's when a root canal becomes necessary (more on this in the next chapter), and many people who had root canals long ago have dead, blackened teeth. When someone gets tired of that dead tooth, he or she can simply cover it with a dental veneer.

With healthy teeth, veneers are especially convenient because they are shaped to the existing tooth, so none of the structure of the tooth has to be removed. This can make teeth look like they have been straightened even without braces or the other straightening techniques discussed in the previous chapter. If a patient has gaps between his or her teeth, veneers can be shaped to fill them.

Finally, with a veneer, a patient will never have to worry about whitening again, because the material of the veneers does not stain at all.

Of course, if you just have one or two veneers, the color of those veneers might end up being undesirable after a long period of time, when the other teeth have become discolored in contrast to the veneer. This brings us back to the solution of whitening, which can help make the surrounding teeth blend with the veneer. However, when we start looking into the true smile makeover, we could be talking about putting veneers on eight teeth at a time. At that point, we really don't have to worry about the color issue anymore.

A lot of celebrities will end up getting their front six teeth done on the top, from canine to canine. Those front teeth end up looking great, but they also stand out, so when they smile it ends up looking like they're missing all but those front teeth—the teeth in the corner of their smile just disappear. So we always recommend that someone who is doing a complete smile makeover place at least eight veneers so that they can fill out that smile corridor and it doesn't look like those teeth have completely disappeared. In some people who have a larger smile, we have to go back to a tenth tooth in order to make sure we get the right result.

We almost always recommend them in even numbers because that way the smile stays balanced. Symmetry in a smile is really important. So we recommend two, four, or eight; and if you do two or four, you have to maintain the whiteness of those surrounding them.

Now, so far, I've only been talking about the top. People can of course also get veneers on their bottom teeth. In particular, for some people, you see the bottom teeth more when they are speaking or smiling. (If you can't picture it, just watch Donald Trump speak sometime.) You can typically get away with only doing six on the bottom.

Again, veneers are a multipurpose solution; however, they are even more powerful as part of an even broader smile makeover, where forms of treatment are mixed and matched. Say you have a wedding coming up and want your smile to look its best—you can start with whitening, followed by a veneer or two; perhaps we even start with Elite Speed Braces if your teeth are out of place, as we did for the bride-to-be in the previous chapter. These treatments can all start building on each other, and before long, you've got a Hollywood smile.

POSITIVE OUTLOOK

"I did everything for my family, and I did nothing for myself while the kids were younger." I've heard this from many people, especially middle-aged and older women. Serena's kids had moved out of the house, and sadly her husband had recently passed away. She had been struggling with the loss of her husband, and she told me she found it hard to smile anymore: "When I do smile, I realize I don't like what people see."

Serena had been born without one of her adult teeth; however, there was no large gap between her teeth. Her other teeth had just moved over to fill in the space. The tooth she was missing was her right lateral incisor—the one next to the front tooth on the top. And her canine or eye tooth—the one that looks like a fang—had moved into its place. Her teeth were otherwise in quite good shape, but she had a pretty noticeable misalignment in this one spot, as well as some small but noticeable gaps between her other teeth on that side due to having one less tooth there.

She had been bullied for it as a child and she wanted to move past the negative effect it had had on her confidence and self-esteem. With veneers, we were able to re-contour the canine tooth into looking like the tooth that was supposed to be there; we did that for the other teeth on that side as well, filling in those spaces between them.

When we finished, it was bittersweet: she made the comment that she wished her husband could see her beautiful smile. At the same time, though, she said she felt like smiling again for the first time since he had passed away. She was grateful, and I was grateful again for the opportunity to profoundly transform someone's outlook on life using the techniques and technology I have spent my career investing in.

PART III

DELIVERING QUALITY DENTAL CARE

CHAPTER 7

NEVER BE REFERRED: HOUSING MULTIPLE SPECIALTIES UNDER ONE ROOF

know the look; I've seen it a thousand times. I say something like, "Johnny needs braces." That's what causes it: the slumped shoulders, the glance at the kids and then back at me. "You mean I have to take this crew to *another* doctor's office?"

One of the goals of my practice is to avoid this by being a one-stop shop for all dental health needs. This means housing multiple specialties under one roof. After all, that's why dentists send you to see other doctors; they're specialists in something else that the dentist can't do. If the dentist could do it himself or herself, he or she certainly isn't going to refer you to another office to have it done.

Our goal is to do absolutely everything under our one roof so that we never have to refer patients out of the office (or at least as seldom as possible). This is good for us as well as for patients, who dislike the inconvenience of having to schlep themselves, and often their families, all over town to go to different appointments. The ideal for a dental practice—and the model I have put in place in my own practice—would be for it to be able to see the kids for pediatric dentistry as well as orthodontics; have all complicated root canals performed in the office by an endodontist; and perform any kind of advanced surgeries, such as the rite of passage for sixteen-year-olds—having their wisdom teeth removed.

WANT TO LEARN MORE ABOUT THE ELITE SMILE EXPERIENCE? CHAPTER 7 COVERS:

- **pediatric dentistry**
- **orthodontics**
- **endodontics**
- **oral surgery**

NOT JUST KIDS' STUFF

Many parents don't realize pediatric dentistry isn't just a niche market; it's a specialization, requiring specific training as well as a kid-friendly environment. Parents need to know that a pediatric dentist can help their kids in a way that a general dentist is not trained to do. If you take your kid to the same dentist you go to, you are actually doing them a disservice.

Most obviously, young children are different from adults in that they still have all or some of their baby teeth. Baby teeth are very different from adult teeth; in particular, they are much more fragile, and the enamel on them is much thinner. For this reason, they are much more susceptible to decay, which can spread from tooth to tooth quickly. Couple this with the fact that kids typically don't take very good care of their teeth, and it turns out that baby teeth need to be attended to much more vigilantly and treated more quickly and decisively when they have problems. Baby teeth aren't as forgiving of neglect as adult teeth are.

Caring for baby teeth may mean fillings, of course, but it also can mean root canals or dental crowns to keep the teeth protected; and, given the size of the teeth, the vast majority of general dentists are not trained to do these procedures. These are the two main procedures that essentially require a pediatric dentist.

Kids tend to be much more fearful of going to the dentist, and pediatric dentists are specially trained to work with the more fearful children. General dentists never receive any training targeted at the psychology of a fearful patient, whereas this is a major part of the pediatric dentist's training. Typically they're trained in sedation as well. So, if the child requires advanced, complex treatment, rather than having to bring the kid in a bunch of times for that experience, we can sedate them to help with the fear, do all the dentistry at once, and then off we go.

Like a lot of professions that involve working with kids, pediatric dentistry tends to attract people of a certain personality type: patient and nurturing, with a positive disposition. These are the kind of people who are naturally good with kids. Couple this with the psychological training pediatric dentists receive to learn how to best work with kids, and it really makes going to the dentist just a vastly better experience for a child when he or she is taken to a pediatric dentist. Incidentally, as part of their psychological training, which general dentists receive none of, pediatric dentists also receive special training to work with patients who have special needs; this is why, typically, if a patient has special needs, they will be referred to a pediatric dentist.

So pediatric dentists play an important role—but so does convenience. This is why I can benefit parents and children among my own patients if I have a pediatric dentist in-house who can serve all of the needs I have just been describing.

IN ALIGNMENT

Having an orthodontist in-house also has benefits that go beyond convenience for the parent—although that is a significant one. The general idea applies to all of the specialists in this chapter, but the orthodontist provides the best illustration of the positive impact of an alignment in approach and philosophy between dentist and orthodontist.

When these two parties are not aligned in this way, conflicts can occur. For example, many orthodontists regularly remove teeth in order to create more space for the others to move around. This could also be done by shaving and contouring some of the teeth or by making the arch bigger, and I see it as an antiquated approach. But still, many orthodontists prefer to remove all four of the first bicuspids (the first premolars, the ones just behind the canines), as they insist that it will have no long-term effect and it frees up space for the orthodontist to work with.

I find removing four healthy teeth to be excessively drastic, and it actually often doesn't go to the root of the problem, because the issue has to do with the airway and the position of the person's bite. I have had several patients come to me with their teeth crowding because of the airway and bite issues, and it turns out they had had their bicuspids removed when they were twelve or thirteen; now they're closer to forty and having the same problem again. Many of these patients who have gotten this "four on the floor" treatment (the bicuspid removal) end up getting migraines or TMJ pain as adults. This means that the removal of the four teeth doesn't adequately address the spacing problem it was introduced to address.

The orthodontist I work with in-house takes a different approach. First, he realizes that airway problems are foundational to problems with bite. Whenever he is planning to put braces on a kid, he first has them get their tonsils and adenoids removed. He only removes teeth in extreme cases where it is absolutely necessary—the moms love to hear this, because they often don't like the idea of having four perfectly healthy teeth removed from their kid's mouth. In cooperation with a dentist, the orthodontist can typically avoid such drastic measures, and some of the treatments I have discussed in previous chapters can be employed instead.

GETTING TO THE ROOT OF THINGS

Another specialist that focuses on an area beyond what most general dentists do, and that dentists regularly have to refer patients to, is the endodontist—a specialist concerned with the *inside* of the tooth.

The part of the tooth that you see, of course, is not the whole tooth. It is also not a living substance; once it is formed, it doesn't grow—it's done. A substantial portion of the tooth, though, is below the surface, making up the root, which is anchored to a ligament that attaches the tooth to the jawbone. The root holds the tooth in place, in addition to being what connects the living, breathing tissue inside the tooth to the rest of the body. This living tissue includes canals containing the nerve and blood vessel of the tooth. The hard outside of the tooth protects this living tissue.

That, of course, is why you have to get numbed up to get dental work done—there's living tissue in there with nerve endings, and it hurts like heck if it's exposed and poked at. This is exactly what happens in the procedure in which the endodontist specializes: the root canal. A root canal requires the endodontist to drill down to expose the canal or canals of the tooth. He or she then uses small files—they actually look and work kind of like little corkscrews—to dig down into the living tissue, or pulp, that fills those canals and dig it out. The endodontist starts with a small file and moves up to progressively larger ones, essentially hollowing the canal out more and more, until finally no pulp is left. The hollow canal is then irrigated with bleach in order to kill off any remaining bacteria down in the canal, which is then filled with a plastic filler.

The tooth is essentially dead at that point. Typically (as I mentioned in the previous chapter), the reason for the root canal in the first place would be that the tooth was dying, and all the dying tissue needs to be removed to prevent infection. To say a tooth is dying is to say that the pulp, the nerve and blood vessel that makes up the living part of the tooth, is decaying. This could be caused by a very large cavity that ended up getting so deep that the bacteria infected the root tissue; or it could be caused by some trauma such as a fall or getting hit in the face. This decay is basically an infection, and at that point the source of the infection needs to be removed. The tooth is generally considered weakened or compromised after a root canal so a crown is placed on top of it to protect it.

Most dentists can do a fairly simple, straightforward root canal. However, an endodontist is required for any more complex cases. An endodontist may also be called in to make a diagnosis on tricky or borderline cases. Finally, there are endodontic surgeries, such as the apicoectomy, that require specific instruments and equipment, as well as a specialization in operating in very small spaces. These, then, can only be done by an endodontist. For all of these reasons, bringing an endodontist in-house cuts down a great deal on the number of referrals a dental office needs to make.

The general dentist is typically used to looking at what is called the clinical crown; the root has a very different structure, which an endodontist is trained to be able to examine and evaluate. For this reason, the endodontist is often better able to diagnose endodontic problems, or at least to confirm a diagnosis. Roots behave a little differently than what we think of as teeth, so you need to have a tooth root specialist. Also, an endodontist typically does root canals pretty much all day every day. I can do root canals, but since it is not my focus and not what I spend most of my time on, I'm not going to be as proficient as an endodontist.

SEEKING WISDOM THROUGH SURGERY

Oral surgery takes several forms, and, as I have mentioned, I specialize in doing one form of oral surgery—namely, tooth removal and implant placement. However, the oral surgeon's bread and butter, which I am unable to do, is the removal of wisdom teeth.

Wisdom teeth make up our third set of molars. The vast majority of people do not have room in their mouths for them to grow in completely (if they grow in at all, as opposed to staying under the surface), so they don't grow to be on the same level as the other molars, and often they crowd the other teeth, which can be painful. Even if someone has room for his or her wisdom teeth, most of the time they will be positioned in such a way that they are very likely to get cavities and have to be removed anyway. Again, they may not grow in enough to be in alignment with the other molars, or they may be rotated in one direction or the other so that their chewing surfaces are not angled properly and don't meet up with the opposing tooth. This makes them useless for chewing, which is our natural way of clearing bacteria out of the crevices in our molars; if the chewing surface of the tooth is not being worked over, then bacteria can tend to gather there and cause cavities. And it's hard to get way back there and brush those guys without gagging.

More often, the wisdom teeth don't have room to come in at all. Rather, they are impacted, meaning they're underneath thin sheets of bone and skin (gum tissue). Basically what has to be done in these cases is that the surgeon has to make an incision in the gum tissue and make sure that tissue is out of the way, then drill through the bone to unhouse the tooth, giving us direct access. This procedure is difficult for several reasons; in particular, it's hard to reach that far back in a person's mouth, and it's difficult to keep the area well-lit and keep all of the things out of the way that need to be kept out of the way (tongue, saliva, gum tissue).

So it's tough—but, fortunately, oral surgeons are trained in this, so it is second nature to them. What this means is that, with an oral surgeon in-house, a dentist will never have to refer a patient out for any kind of tooth removal. That dental office will be able to remove any teeth that need removed no matter how complex the procedure to do so.

Oral surgeons can also correct major jaw alignment problems that cannot be addressed by traditional orthodontics. In these cases, the bottom jaw (or, in rarer and more complex cases, the upper jaw) needs to be reset. This elaborate procedure, known as orthognathic surgery, takes a team of specialists, including of course an oral surgeon—that is a level of surgical complexity that takes special training.

Now, doesn't it seem so much better to have that team of specialists all in one place than to have to bounce from office to office? The orthodontist (who would typically be the one to prescribe this surgery) can communicate directly with the oral surgeon, telling him or her exactly how the jaw needs to repositioned, and the oral surgeon simply carries out what the orthodontist recommends. While the oral surgeon executes the play, so to speak, the orthodontist acts as his or her coach, and it is obviously preferable to have them together in the same room.

These doctors communicate with one another every day, whereas in typical cases they wouldn't communicate with each other directly at all except for the occasional phone call, where they have to play phone tag, or email, which can take forever to get a response to. They can actually examine the patient together, rather than one doctor trying to explain a complex diagnosis over the phone. Again, this type of alignment is a major benefit of keeping these different specialties in-house, and it goes far beyond the convenience of not having to go to multiple offices—though of course that is still a benefit.

Oral surgeons also provide an added benefit. Within the last decade, more and more of them are spending two years of their six-year oral surgery program getting their medical license. Not only are they graduating as dentists, but now they are medical doctors as well and will thus be able to treat any potential complications that could possibly arise during dental procedures. They would be called in, for instance, to work with a patient who is medically compromised or has some type of severe medical problems. They are also all trained in sedation, so the expertise needed for sedation dentistry is built into the oral surgeon's resume.

A TEAM EFFORT

When doctors are housed together in a single practice, they will (or should) have a unified philosophy about how to go about treating things. The fact is that there are many different approaches to dentistry and oral health, and this can be a source of frustration to parents in particular.

Having the team all on hand also just has the obvious benefit of … well, having the team all on hand. For example, being in St. Augustine, Florida, we get a lot of walk-in patients from out of town; they don't have access to their usual dentist, so the more we can offer without having to send them all over town the better. Recently, a boy came in that required a real all-hands-on-deck situation. He had been at the beach, playing on a boogie board, when he slipped in the water and the boogie board popped straight up and hit him directly in the face, breaking one of his front teeth.

Half of the tooth was broken off, and the part that remained was loose, as were a few other teeth in the front of his mouth that had suffered the impact of the boogie board; so we stabilized the teeth with orthodontic wires. The break had exposed the nerve, so the traumatized tooth required a root canal. Finally, we needed to craft a partial crown to restore it to its original shape as well as to further stabilize and protect what remained of the tooth. This took a few hours, and he came in right before we closed, so the team stayed after hours to help him.

His family was in town from New Jersey, and it was the first day of his family's vacation. If we hadn't had the orthodontist and endodontist there to work on his tooth, not to mention the CEREC technology that allowed us to craft a partial crown for him right on the spot, he would likely have had to be rushed home for an emergency root canal, cutting the family vacation short. He was also in severe pain and would be until that root canal, so the trip home would not have been fun either. The way we had it arranged, though, we were able to get him in and out in a relatively short time, and his family was able to resume the vacation.

Unfortunately, this is not the typical approach—which is why the frustrated reaction of parents who have to take their kids all over town is so well known. Dentists often see other doctors in the field of oral health as somehow in competition with them—especially, of course, other dentists. Why would they want to bring others into the same office with them? I have a totally different mind-set: bringing other doctors under my umbrella is all I want to do. This way, I have built my practice to have all the advantages and skill sets of both the general dentist and multiple specialists.

CHAPTER 8

PATIENT CARE AND CUSTOMER SATISFACTION

vividly remember one night at my office: it was storming outside, and it was very cold—well, at least it was what counts as "very cold" in Florida. My practice, Elite Smiles, had only been open for a few months. I was just saying goodbye to the last of our patients for the day when the storm knocked out the power to our building.

Perfect timing, right? I mean, we were done for the day. Our patient, however, was bound to a wheelchair, and my office was located on the second floor. There was no generator in the building, so the elevator was not operating. Our patient wouldn't be going anywhere until the power came back on.

Coincidentally, the practice had been given a candle set as a sort of office-warming gift, so we quickly set our consultation room aglow. We called the patient's wife, who was nearby, and she joined us at the office. We sat talking for a while as we waited for the power to come back on, and eventually we all got hungry. My wife delivered dinner and a bottle of wine, and she and I dined with this other couple by candlelight, and we learned all about them—about their children, who were grown; about why they moved to St. Augustine; and about their life together.

> *My practice is part of my community, which includes many wonderful people. Our task is to serve those people with the highest-quality dental care we can.*

The power came back on just as we were pouring the last of the wine, and we were soon seeing our guests off. That unexpected evening has shaped the core values of my practice; to this day, I see my patients as guests, and that is how we refer to them in the office. What that night means to me now is that my practice is part of my community, which includes many wonderful people. Our task is to serve those people with the highest-quality dental care we can.

As you may suspect after reading this book, we at my practice see the role of dental care in people's lives somewhat differently than the average dental practice—especially in the current world of corporate-owned practices. This chapter digs into this difference of approach.

- **the dental care experience**

- **the corporate dentistry takeover**

- **dental anxiety**

- **practice culture**

- **patient education**

"YOU WIN WITH PEOPLE"

Have you ever seen someone post on Facebook about his or her great experience at the dentist's office? Most likely not. I wish it happened more often, but the truth is that standing out from the crowd in the dental field is not easy. A filling is a filling; a cleaning is pretty much the same from one dentist to the next; and no one gets excited about either one.

Like any business, though, we want raving fans; we want our patients to actually enjoy going to the dentist. At the end of the day, we want them to walk away with something more than the tooth-colored filling in their mouth. So how does a dental practice turn its patients into raving fans?

As an Ohio State football fan, I learned a lot of lessons early on from Hall of Fame former coach Woody Hayes. One of those lessons particularly sticks with me; he once said, "You win with people." This captures my "people first" approach to my dental practice and has become my company motto. As I mentioned, I see my patients as guests, and we strive to treat them that way. This is also reflected in our statement of core values:

1. **Fun:** Enjoy what you are doing and make the process fun for those around you.

2. **Positive:** Focus on what you can control, and help lift others up.

3. **Learn:** Be coachable, be willing to learn, and have a desire to teach others.

4. **Integrity:** Stand behind our work and provide elite treatment.

My approach, then, has been to focus on the level of personal care and attention guests get when they are being treated. Thinking of dental care as involving a customer service aspect is key to creating the kind of guest experience I aim for. Take an example from another industry: a restaurant that is not competing on price with the big corporate fast-food chains had better deliver a high-quality customer service experience, because without it that business will die. No one will have a reason to go there.

The restaurants that are succeeding today are either the lowest priced or are offering exemplary customer service. Even the big corporate chains, Chick-Fil-A for instance, can have a slightly higher price point, but customers see it as worthwhile not only because they like the product but also because the service is remarkable. They are willing to pay more for the better experience.

A similar development is happening in contemporary dentistry, especially when it comes to the low-priced option. The baby boomer dentists we are used to are starting to retire, and young dentists are coming out of dental school with massive debt burdens, so they don't have the capacity to buy out older practices or start their own. Instead, corporations are buying all of the offices and staffing them with these young dentists. This leads to a sort of "corporate dentistry takeover," where practices are run more and more with attention only to the bottom line. Prices are driven down, but these practices breed a factory-like mentality in young dentists, who have to hit quotas for how many patients they get in and out of the office on a daily basis. (A similar development has more obviously taken place in medicine, with the fall of the family doctor in private practice and the rise of doctors contracting solely with hospitals or corporate medical groups.)

> *A corporate dentistry model moves us away from a patient-centered approach and toward treating patients more like numbers than like people.*

A corporate dentistry model moves us away from a patient-centered approach and toward treating patients more like numbers than like people. A corporate practice is also not likely to take the intensive, holistic approach to dental health and care that I encourage in this book. A successful practice, on the other hand, should do all it can to buck these trends, refocusing on the experience that the patient has. In other words, bring a customer service focus to dentistry, and strive to go above and beyond in that department.

ELITE CARE AND COMFORT

Believe me, your dentist knows that a lot of people have anxiety about going to the dentist; some people are even terrified. The best dental practices are sensitive to this and take measures to respond to this anxiety and make the dental visit as comfortable and stress-free as possible.

At the time of this writing, I am in the process of constructing a new space for my practice. Part of my aim at the new location is for the patient to feel like he or she is not even at a dental office from the moment he or she walks in the door. Instead, the office has a warm, inviting, coffee-shop feel, with a lot of open space, natural light, and high ceilings.

At Elite Smiles, patients are greeted as they come in by a host or hostess at a stand rather than a receptionist behind a desk; and they are led either straight to a private chair or, if there is a short wait, to an actual coffee shop located inside the office, where they can get coffee or even a sandwich or pastry from a small kitchen. Because I see all of the patients in my practice as guests, my staff and I try to treat them that way, from the moment they first walk in the door. We even offer small gifts to our new patients. We give larger gifts as prizes in a quarterly drawing that patients can enter as a thank-you for being loyal patients or sending referrals our way. We also try to accommodate the different needs of our patients. For parents, we even provide a playground area to keep the kids entertained during visits.

Once a patient is in his or her chair—which is in a private space—a member of my "Happiness Team" (staff who are focused on the patient experience) visits him or her to discuss the purpose of the visit, what procedures will be done, and any goals or concerns the patient might have.

This visit serves two purposes: first, it is a key component of patient education. Second, it is an aspect of relieving patient fear or anxiety. Often what frightens us is just the unknown, and transparently laying everything on the table regarding what is going to happen during the visit can alleviate that fear.

Changing the environment of the dental office is another way of addressing anxiety and fear. Often, patients associate certain sounds and smells with the dentist's office. It's never pleasant to have to hear the whirring drill being used down the hall when you are waiting to see the dentist. At Elite Smiles, we broadcast soothing white noise and offer noise-cancelling headphones that filter out the frequencies of the drill or of conversations going on next door.

We also have a scent machine hooked up to the air handler in the office, so that a pleasant scent comes through the vents, not only masking any potential odors from the dental equipment but actually establishing a calmer, more inviting atmosphere. Just to give you an idea of how far removed from a dental office this small touch can make you feel: we use the same scent machine as the one used in the Ritz-Carlton.

Research even went into choosing the paint colors for the new office. We are not just putting up whatever colors I find pleasing; rather, we are using soothing blues, greens, and greys that studies have shown produce a calming effect.

> *All of these touches not only provide a patient experience very different from the one patients will find down the street or around the corner, but they also help to put nervous or fearful patients at ease.*

All of these touches not only provide a patient experience very different from the one patients will find down the street or around the corner, but they also help to put nervous or fearful patients at ease. Finally, for patients who are so terrified at the prospect of a dental visit that all of these measures are inadequate, we have the option of sedation dentistry; either via a pill or an IV, a patient can receive a sedative that allows them to just go to sleep. When they wake, the dental visit is over; any work they might have needed done is done. This option works best for people with acute anxiety.

SHAPING THE PRACTICE

Building a practice that is responsive to the anxieties and fears of patients requires effort and investment, but the effort and investment are worthwhile from a customer service standpoint. High-quality customer service in the dental space requires effort and investment to be devoted to the staffing and culture of a practice. It also demands that similar importance be granted to the practice's capabilities, obtainable through continuing training and technological investment.

> *Effort and investment are worthwhile from a customer service standpoint.*

My staff are committed to the highest standard of care; we reinforce this commitment through the culture of the practice, which we build through hiring, shape by encouraging employees to bond with one another through social activities, and motivate with a purpose-driven attitude.

In hiring, many dentists get lost in the questions of qualifications and experience, looking for staff with fancy credentials. This may help in the factory-like corporate practice, but if the aim is patient happiness, the questions of values and personality are more important. Skills can be taught to employees who are open to learning them. For instance, when one of my employees started out, she had been a bartender and had just finished dental assisting school. She was inexperienced, but her work ethic and positive attitude were obvious. She is now an office manager and a very valued employee.

Social science research has shown that members of the millennial generation are mission-driven; they want the work they do in life to be contributing to some greater good. A large portion of my staff is made up of young women of this generation, and we try to build a culture that reminds them that they are pursuing a larger purpose beyond just coming in to get a paycheck. Given the importance of dental care to people's overall health, the work they do is important and can profoundly help the many people they encounter on a day-to-day basis.

We also pursue initiatives that build culture beyond the day-to-day. For example, every time we get a new referral, we set aside twenty-five dollars to fund a mission trip to the Dominican Republic, where we offer free dental care. When we have adequate funding, the staff can participate in this mission, which instills a sense of the higher purpose of the practice and the value of the work that we do. It incentivizes the staff to do quality work day in and day out—and not just because they could get a free trip to the Dominican Republic. They really value the opportunity to provide their services to people who typically would not have access to it.

Every time we get a new referral, we set aside twenty-five dollars to fund a mission trip to the Dominican Republic, where we offer free dental care.

As I mentioned, I have a "Happiness Team"—staff who are devoted to the customer service side of things. I call our head of internal marketing the "Happiness Coordinator" because it is her responsibility to make people in the office happy by getting patient feedback, monitoring our reviews to ensure that they are positive, and soliciting and tracking referrals. At the end of the day, though, the only way you can get those things is if you provide a top-notch experience. One aspect of that is staying on the cutting edge regarding the techniques and technologies that are available to a dental practice.

My staff and I both participate regularly in continuing education. If a practice does not do this, then it will lag behind in providing the best possible care for patients. So, training for the entire office is something that we really stress and is really important to us. On a similar note, I make sure my practice has the highest quality and most up-to-date technology, equipment, and customer service facilities. Our equipment is state of the art. This is an investment, of course— as is the continuing education—but ultimately it is an investment in the practice's ability to provide the best care possible and serve the community as well as we can.

THE "WHY" BEHIND YOUR DENTAL TREATMENT

I often tell the story of the mother who is showing her son how to cook a roast in the oven. She cuts the roast into two wide pieces and places them side-by-side. The son asks why she does this, and the mother says, "That was the way my mother taught me to do it. I'll ask her if she knows why." They call up Grandma, who says, "My oven when I was growing up was too small to fit the whole roast in. So I cut it in half to put it in two pans so it would fit in the oven. But your oven is bigger; there's no reason for you to keep doing that."

Oddly enough, I think this story applies to dentistry; many patients come in and get their dental treatment without thinking about or understanding the purpose of the procedures they are getting done. However, it is important to me that patients and staff alike understand the "why" of what we do for them. Communicating that clearly to the patient enables us to make sure that everyone's— both patient's and dentist's—expectations are aligned and that we are pursuing the right treatment for that patient.

We have many avenues of communication for keeping in touch with our patients. We also have digital imaging tools that we can use to actually show them what effect various treatments will have—or, in some cases, what negative effects *not* getting treatment may have. Patients should be able to understand what their expectations should be, what's going to happen during a procedure, and what happens next. As I mentioned, this knowledge can also do a lot to put the anxious patient at ease.

It is also important to educate patients in general about the importance of oral health overall. This is a large part of why I am writing this book, in fact. I also provide my patients with a newsletter, which serves to maintain patient loyalty but also guides patients who are craving information about dental health to my practice and my website—which is chock-full of information, including videos and blog posts—instead of to the wider internet, where information is unreliable.

Education, then, is the final component of the patient-centered approach that we follow at Elite Smiles. We go the distance to ensure that every aspect of a patient's visit is of the best quality it can be. This starts with our VIP treatment. Rather than just bells and whistles, we have included these aspects into our practice in order to make each patient as comfortable—and relaxed—as possible. We then follow this with the substance of dental work provided by a skilled and knowledgeable staff that uses the latest technology to ensure the best possible results. We then educate our patients so that they can continue the work of dental care on their own. The process, as we see it, is critical to achieving the best results: happy guests who just might come away having enjoyed being at the dentist.

CHAPTER 9

THE GROWTH OF ELITE DENTAL CARE

was very excited the first time I heard my name read out over a loudspeaker: "Steve Freeman, you just won the train set!" This was at a model train show my father took me to when I was a kid. It was the first time I had ever won anything. It was also my first train set; but after that, my father and I spent a lot of time together building model railroads and model scenery for the backdrop. I once broke off a piece of my front tooth trying to pry apart two pieces of track that were stuck together by biting on one of them. That was one of my first lessons from my oral surgeon father: "Teeth are not tools."

This is just one respect in which I enjoyed working with my hands as a kid; I also did a lot of art projects. But the projects where I worked together with my father influenced me particularly strongly. As I got older, in addition to building models with him, I started working with my father in his office, even sometimes assisting him in emergency cases. It fascinated me and I enjoyed it. Still, I wasn't ready to consider a career in dentistry yet. I wanted to forge my own path, and, like many ambitious young men, I pushed back against the idea of doing anything like what my father had done.

Still, my passion for working with my hands, coupled with my desire to be my own boss and my drive to fix problems when I encountered them, eventually led me back to a career as a dentist. In this chapter I finish outlining my vision for elite dental care by discussing my own growth as a dentist and how it led me into the realms of entrepreneurship and then coaching other dentists. The appeal of dentistry for me lay in the opportunity to help people be healthier. The growth of my business and my coaching of other dentists simply spreads this opportunity to an ever-larger group of people.

WANT TO LEARN MORE ABOUT THE ELITE SMILE EXPERIENCE? CHAPTER 9 COVERS:

- **my growth as a dentist**
- **my growth as an entrepreneur**
- **my growth as a coach**

MY OWN BOSS

I've never been very good at being told what to do. Knowing that about myself led me to realize that working for myself, being my own boss, was a top career priority. I likewise have always had the entrepreneurial spirit. I remember talking to my sister when I was young about all of the companies I would create when I grew up. "You can't do all that!" she would say. Of course, this just made me more determined; it emboldened me to go ahead and do what she said I couldn't. I guess I owe her a "thank you" in that case. (Incidentally, she is an entrepreneur herself. I guess it runs in the family.)

I knew that one of the things I was looking for in a career was that I wanted to set my own schedule. This is partly due to witnessing the example of my father. While he had his own oral surgery practice, his bread and butter was removing the wisdom teeth of teenagers. This meant that his busiest times of the year were when school was out; of course, that was also when my sister and I were out of school. His work schedule prevented us from being able to really take vacations. I wanted more leeway to spend time with my family.

As for the type of work I wanted to do, I dabbled with the idea of working in real estate, and thought also about becoming a teacher. From the point of view of being your own boss, though, being a teacher is certainly a no-go, and the frantic schedule of a real estate agent sounded awful to me.

At one point I was seriously considering medical school, but general medicine left me cold. Here, another aspect of my personality, related to my passion for working with my hands, plays a role. If I find a problem, I'm not satisfied with finding someone else to take care of it if I can take care of it myself. Think about what the general practitioner or family physician does: he or she acquires information about the patient; comes to a conclusion or diagnosis based on their years of education and experience; and lays out a plan, writes a prescription, or makes a referral to a specialist. Actually carrying out the treatment is up to someone else, whether it be a patient taking his or her medication or a surgeon making an intervention.

As for the assessment and diagnosis part, much the same happens with dentistry; however, when an intervention needs to be made, the dentist is typically the one that actually does it. If a patient has a cavity, guess what? I can clean out the cavity, fill it, and off we go. It is much more hands-on; in that respect, dentists have more in common with surgeons than they do with general physicians. I wanted a job like that, where, if I found a problem, I could fix it, rather than just telling someone else how to fix it.

So I just kept being pulled back to dentistry; I already had some familiarity with it, of course, through my father's oral surgery practice. I actually remember the day I decided that that would be the direction I would take. My girlfriend (now wife) and I were in the car, talking about our plans for the future, and it just suddenly seemed clear which direction I should go; I said, "That's it. I'm going to dental school." My plan was to finish dental school and an oral surgery residency just as my father was retiring, so I could take over his practice.

And that is exactly what happened. As a huge Ohio State football fan (my dad played football for legendary coach Woody Hayes, whom I quoted in the previous chapter), I was thrilled to be able to go to the very prestigious dental school there. At first, I wanted to specialize in oral surgery, but I quickly became more interested in cosmetic procedures, especially as this avenue of work would give me a great deal of control over my schedule.

After finishing dental school, I opened my practice in 2008 focused mainly on cosmetic dentistry. This turned out to be bad timing; right around 2008 was exactly when, suddenly, no one could afford cosmetic dental procedures anymore! I shifted gears to general dentistry and focused more on affordability. As a generalist, though, I was worried about becoming a jack of all trades and master of none. I wanted to really dig into a specialty and hone my craft. I also kept seeing problems that I thought I should be able to fix—from obstructive sleep disorders to people with missing teeth who were putting extra stress on their other teeth.

As I saw these recurring problems, I kept extending my areas of proficiency so that I could treat them. In the process, I kept feeling drawn back to the type of oral surgery that my father had practiced, and I eventually took advanced training in order to be able to place dental implants. The implant is now my specialty, the craft I am an expert in. It is in the realm of tooth replacement that I felt, and still feel, like I can have the greatest impact.

This focus has allowed me to grow my practice in order to be able to bring other doctors with other specialties into the office. With the help of these other doctors, I am able to serve more people in my community and serve them better than I would otherwise be able to. I am now at a point where, as I mentioned previously, the practice is moving into a new, larger space.

At the same time, in the process of bringing other dentists into the practice, I began to develop a passion for playing an educational role for other dentists. I wanted to see how many people I could actually help have a great experience in the dental office. This of course led me to focus heavily on the customer service of my own practice, but I also wanted to reach people beyond the bounds of my community. I set out on a new path of consulting and coaching other dentists so that they could bring the type of experience offered at Elite Smiles to their own communities. This book is the next step in that attempt to have a broader influence through educating not only patients but other dentists as well.

IMPROVING DENTISTRY

While I love the hands-on part of dentistry, my own work directly with patients has lately been replaced more and more by my role as a coach, both within my practice and outside its walls. At the office, I play the role of a kind of cheerleader for my team, in addition to making sure that the systems and processes the practice relies on are running smoothly. I also make sure, in order to ensure the highest level of patient care, that all of my staff are on the same page and up to date in their technological know-how, their professional dental terminology, and their individual roles within the big choreographed performance that takes place on a daily basis at Elite Smiles.

My practice is big enough that I have a strong leadership team to take care of much of the staff coaching, but I devote a lot of time to coaching the coaches. I have also started a second business coaching dentists outside my practice. Rather than focusing on continuing education on techniques or procedures, I teach these dentists about business development and how they can spread the same type of customer experience throughout the profession by creating other great offices across the country. The better the patient experience, the better and more fun dental care is for everyone. So, as a coach, I'm focused on spreading the fun in the dental profession, as opposed to spreading the ability to do a filling better.

Passing on this type of knowledge is now what I most want to do in my career. As I mentioned earlier, teaching was an early interest of mine, and I considered a career in teaching but decided the bureaucracy of the education system was too confining for me. I have now carved out a place for myself where I get to teach my own passion to others on an advanced level and in my own terms. In my coaching and consulting business, I do monthly coaching calls with other dentists. I have products, such as DVDs and other educational material, available to dentists to help them grow their practices; basically, I just want to provide insight into how I've grown my own practice so that others can follow that example.

A COMMON MISTAKE

In my experience in coaching, the problem I have run into most often is what I would call overspecialization. Of course, specialization is important and can be very good for a dental practice; I don't mean to deny that. After all, a major part of my journey, and my success, was my eventual specialization in implants. This gave me a particular niche to cater to. However, while I was specializing in this way, I was also working to ensure that my practice had all of the other capabilities that might be demanded of it.

> *Making a niche service into the whole of your practice is a great example of putting all of your eggs in one basket. The niche or the specialty is not incompatible with the general practice.*

In other words, making a niche service into the whole of your practice is a great example of putting all of your eggs in one basket. The niche or the specialty is not incompatible with the general practice. There is no reason that you can't provide every dental service under one roof; and, in fact, being able to promote your specialized niche is even more effective when it is against this background of the general practice.

A dental practice is, after all, a business. Thinking about it from this point of view, different areas of dentistry and different specialized procedures can be seen as different revenue streams, and if one revenue stream starts to dry up, it is better to be able to open the valve on another one than to be left with no other options. Diversifying the practice thus means being able to be more flexible, to be more nimble in response to the market, and to stay balanced when changes in the market occur.

I learned this lesson the hard way myself, of course, during the financial crisis of 2008. My practice at the time specialized in cosmetic procedures, but when the market for cosmetic procedures dropped off completely, I had to be nimble enough to move in a different direction, regain my footing, and continue to grow my practice. If I hadn't had that flexibility, I would no longer have a practice.

Staying up-to-date on new techniques and technology is a core aspect of being able to stay on top of changes in the market. This also illustrates to patients that the practice is willing to invest in high-quality patient care. These new technologies, like CEREC and some of the others I have mentioned in this book, tend to make providing care more convenient for the dentist and for the patient— they typically make appointments faster, easier, and more enjoyable. Finally, as certain techniques become obsolete or certain markets start to dry up, investing in techniques and technology allows a practice that flexibility to move to something new.

By providing advice and encouragement, I hope I can help other dentists be successful. In doing so, I will be able to reach more patients indirectly than I ever would be able to actually see in my office. Of course, at the same time, I remain devoted to my own practice; here also, though, the biggest value I think I can bring is in coaching others—making sure that everyone is focused on the right thing: not just the procedure or getting patients in and out but the overall experience that the patient is having. That way, I can have the greatest possible positive effect on the oral health—and thus the overall health—of the members of my community.

CONCLUSION

n this book I have emphasized the importance of dental health and dental care in a lot of ways. In some ways, this is an uphill battle: people tend to see dentistry as less serious than other branches of medicine—that is, if they recognize it as a branch of medicine at all! Many see it as merely cosmetic or as involving nothing more than the simplistic procedure of cleaning people's teeth on a regular basis and telling them to brush and floss.

The reality is that taking care of the health of your mouth is incredibly important; the condition of your teeth is more than a cosmetic concern. The health of your mouth plays a major role in affecting your overall bodily health.

But the reality is that taking care of the health of your mouth is incredibly important; the condition of your teeth is more than a cosmetic concern. The health of your mouth plays a major role in affecting your overall bodily health. Given the interconnections between oral health, the immune system, and other bodily systems, it is safe to say that a good smile can literally be a life-saver.

You could even say this about cosmetic dental procedures, which, as I have discussed, can have a major impact on self-confidence and psychological health. Some of them also do double duty by having a potential effect on bodily health as well; for instance, implants can prevent many of the negative health effects of missing teeth, and in some cases straightening teeth can improve sleep by affecting the airway.

> *Having a diversified practice can also make the process much more convenient—the patient can get everything they need done under one roof.*

Of course, I know that many people in my potential audience avoid the dentist out of fear or due to bad experiences they have had at a dental office, whether as kids or even more recently. It's this issue that brings the investment in customer service to the forefront of my approach: There are new techniques and technologies that can make the dental care experience faster, easier, safer, and more comfortable. Having a diversified practice can also make the process much more convenient—the patient can get everything they need done under one roof. People have hectic lives in our society, and making dental care easily accessible is a key aspect of providing it to the community.

Helping people *smile to live* and contributing to the community is the overall aim of what I do, and of everything I have discussed in this book. I have been fortunate to have a strong and wonderful community in my city, and I hope to continue to grow that community through coaching other dentists to adopt my patient-focused approach to dental care, as well as through the lessons that I hope this book delivers to readers, whether dentist or patient.

OUR SERVICES

Elite Smiles offers a full range of services help you achieve and maintain a healthy smile. Our experienced dentists provide comprehensive dentistry in Saint Augustine, Florida and the surrounding areas. When you visit our practice, you can expect our dentists and team to be attentive to your needs, giving you their full attention and providing you with an open, home-like atmosphere in which you can feel at ease. Our office features the latest technologies, including 3D cone beam imaging and same-day CEREC dental crowns, to make your experience as convenient and comfortable as possible and ensure that your treatments are tailored precisely to your needs.

Our services include:

- Dental Implant & Crown
- Cosmetic Dentistry
    - Dental Veneers
    - Smile Makeovers
    - Invisalign®
    - Elite Speed Braces

- General Dentistry
  - Deep Dental Cleanings
  - Dental Implants
  - Infinite Teeth Whitening
  - Dentures
  - Live Denture Free
  - Same Day Dental Crowns
  - Sleep Apnea & Snoring Treatment
  - Tooth Sensitivity & Grinding

- Dental Technology
  - 3D Cone Beam Imaging
  - Intraoral Cameras
  - CEREC
  - Digital X-Rays

We keep our focus on you and your needs and pay close attention to detail to ensure that you receive beautiful, long-lasting solutions for your smile. We are committed to meeting your oral health needs in a friendly and comfortable environment. Elite Smiles has been featured on NBC, ABC, CBS, Channel 4 Television, and First Coast Magazine. For more information about our services, our dentists, and to make an appointment, please visit www.elitesmilesdentistry.com.